D1724358

Treatment of Renal Anemia with Recombinant Human Erythropoietin

Contributions to Nephrology
Vol. 66

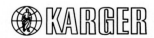

Basel · München · Paris · London · New York · New Delhi · Singapore · Tokyo · Sydney

International Workshop, Wolfenbüttel, November 22–24, 1987

Treatment of Renal Anemia with Recombinant Human Erythropoietin

Volume Editors
K. M. Koch, K. Kühn, B. Nonnast-Daniel, Hannover;
P. Scigalla, Mannheim

76 figures and 41 tables, 1988

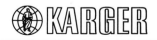 KARGER

Basel · München · Paris · London · New York · New Delhi · Singapore · Tokyo · Sydney

Contributions to Nephrology

Library of Congress Cataloging-in-Publication Data
Treatment of renal anemia with recombinant human erythropoietin.
(Contributions to nephrology; vol. 66)
'International workshop, Wolfenbüttel, November 22–24, 1987.'
Includes bibliographies and index.
1. Renal anemia – Chemotherapy – Congresses.   2. Erythropoietin – Therapeutic use –
Congresses   I. Koch, K. M.   II. Series: Contributions to nephrology; v. 66.
[DNLM: 1. Anemia – therapy – congresses.   2. Erythropoietin – therapeutic use – congresses.
3. Kidney Diseases – complications – congresses.   W1 CO778UN v. 66/WJ 300 T784 1987]
RC641.7.R44T74 1988   616.1'32061   88-6808
ISBN 3–8055–4764–1

Bibliographic Indices
This publication is listed in bibliographic services, including Current Contents®
and Index Medicus.

Contents

Contents

Multicenter Trial of Recombinant Human Erythropoietin: Special Studies

Preface

This volume of *Contributions to Nephrology* reports on a workshop on the 'Treatment of Renal Anemia with Recombinant Human Erythropoietin', which took place in November 1987 in the Herzog August Bibliothek in Wolfenbüttel. The workshop's title impresses as a straightforward clinical therapeutical topic, but indirectly it also addresses many achievements of research in biological sciences and clinical medicine: There are the decades of intelligent and untiring basic research which culminated in the availability of highly purified erythropoietin and almost complete knowledge of the chemical structure of this hormone. This was the prerequisite for the application of the tools of modern molecular biology to the task of producing recombinant human erythropoietin. In an amazingly short period of time these efforts were crowned by success and now sufficient amounts of the recombinant hormone are available to be used safely in the treatment of renal anemia. Parallel to these scientific developments there was equally successful research in the physiology and pathophysiology of erythropoietin. Today we are very near to the exact localization of the site of erythropoietin production within the kidney and we understand the role of erythropoietin deficiency in the pathogenesis of renal anemia.

All these exciting developments were covered in the first part of the workshop. We were very fortunate to have assembled for this purpose a group of leading scientists from various fields of erythropoietin research. The second and third parts of the workshop were devoted to the evaluation of the results of the application of recombinant human erythropoietin in the treatment of renal anemia. The reports are derived from the experiences in a multicenter trial of recombinant human erythropoietin in patients with terminal renal failure sponsored by Boehringer Mannheim. But clinical experience in this workshop was not limited to our multicenter trial alone. We are very grateful that also leading clinicians engaged in earlier trials with recombinant human erythropoietin followed our invitation. By having them at the workshop together with all the basic scientists we intended to provide sufficient critical mass for thourough evaluation of our results. I hope that this intention is reflected in the discussion parts of this volume.

The results of the multicenter trial clearly demonstrate that human recombinant erythropoietin is an effective therapeutical tool. At future meetings of this kind, when more data from long-term experience are available, it will be decided whether we covered all benefits but also all adverse effects of the recombinant hormone.

I thank Boehringer Mannheim for sponsoring this workshop and the staff of S. Karger AG for all their effort and help, which ensured timely completion of this volume. Finally I am very much indebted to Prof. Dr. R. Raabe for admitting the workshop to the Augusteerhalle of the Herzog August Bibliothek. I believe that all of us during the meeting felt obliged to the spiritus loci and enjoyed to spend two days of scientific exchange within this unique institution.

K. M. Koch

Contr. Nephrol., vol. 66, pp. 1–16 (Karger, Basel 1988)

Regulation of Erythropoietin Production

Armin Kurtz, Kai-Uwe Eckardt, Lesley Tannahill, Christian Bauer

Physiologisches Institut der Universität Zürich, Switzerland

Erythropoietin (EPO) is the primary humoral regulator of erythropoiesis. Its function is to stimulate the proliferation and differentiation of erythroid precursor cells. Since the discovery by Carnot and Deflandre [1] in 1906 of an humoral factor that stimulates erythropoiesis, EPO behaved as a somewhat elusive hormone for more than eight decades. Not only the structure of the molecule was subject to speculation but also the regulation and mode of its biogenesis. Three theories have been advanced in the past to explain the generation of EPO. First, a plasma enzyme generates EPO from a precursor molecule produced in the kidney [2], second, a renal enzyme splits EPO from a precursor present in the plasma [3] and third, EPO is directly synthesized. Now we know the structure of the molecule [4, 6], the sequence of its mRNA [6–8] and the organs containing mRNA for EPO [9, 10]. On the basis of this information it can be inferred that EPO is directly synthesized by the fetal liver and by the adult kidney. This conclusion confirms the concepts that the liver is the main production site during fetal life [11] and that the kidneys produce almost 90% of the EPO in adult mammals [12, 13]. The regulation and physiological impact of fetal EPO production is only poorly understood. Therefore, we will focus on *renal* EPO production, whereby in consideration of the knowledge presently available we will present and discuss our own results.

Materials and Methods

Animals. Male SIV strain rats (250–280 g) or male ICR strain mice (28–32 g) were used for all experiments except studies on the effect of polycythemia on EPO response, where female ICR strain mice were used.

Normobaric Hypoxia and Functional Anemia. Animals were exposed to oxygen-depleted (13.5, 10.5 or 8% O_2) or carbon monoxide-enriched (0.1% CO) atmospheres using incubation chambers that were gassed with a mixture of normal air and nitrogen or carbon monoxide.

Experiments with Polycythemic Animals. Mice were rendered polycythemic during a 15-day period of intermittent (20–22 h/day) normobaric hypoxia (7–8% O_2). Four and 12 days later, groups of 5 polycythemic animals together with normocythemic controls were exposed to either (i) hypoxic hypoxia (8% O_2) for 3 h or (ii) carbon monoxide (0.1%) for 3 h or (iii) treated with cobalt chloride (60 mg/kg s. c.) for 12 h and bled thereafter for determination of hematocrit and serum EPO levels.

Experiments with Diuretics. One of four diuretic drugs was injected into mice prior to a hypoxic eposure: acetazolamide (25 mg/kg), furosemide (20 mg/kg), hydrochlorothiazide (6 mg/kg) or amiloride (2 mg/kg). The natriuretic effect of these drugs was estimated by collecting the urine voided by 5 animals each within 3 h and measuring the respective Na content by flame photometry.

Hypobaric Hypoxia in Man. Six healthy male volunteers were exposed to a simulated altitude of 4,000 m (0.61 atm) for 5 h using a decompression chamber.

Assays for EPO. Radioimmunoassay (RIA) for EPO was performed as described [14], using a rabbit antiserum derived against human recombinant EPO and iodinated recombinant EPO (Amersham Lab., UK) as tracer. In brief, 100 µl of samples plus 20 µl of 30% BSA were incubated with 100 µl of antiserum (1/90,000) for 24 h. 100 µl of tracer (8×10^{-11} mol/l ^{125}I EPO) were then added and after an additional incubation period of 24 h separation of free and bound ligand carried out using a second antibody technique. Because of different immunoreactivity of human, mouse and rat EPO with the antiserum, species-specific standards were used: (i) the 2nd International Reference Preparation (IRP) of human urinary EPO (WHO) for determinations of human samples; EPO-enriched serum pools of (ii) mice and (iii) rats for determinations in these species (fig. 1). Pools were prepared by exposing animals to normobaric hypoxia for 18 h and the respective EPO content then calibrated in vivo against human EPO (2nd IRP). A modification of the exhypoxic polycythemic mouse *bioassay* [15] using intermittent normobaric hypoxia (7–8% O_2, 20–22 h/day for 14 days) for induction of polycythemia [14] was used for these in vivo determinations.

Northern Blot Analysis. Total RNA was extracted from whole-kidney homogenates using the guanidinium-cesium chloride method [16]; mRNA was selected by oligo(dT)-cellulose chromatography [17]. mRNA samples (20 µg) were denatured in formamide/formaldehyde and electrophoresed in a 1.0% agarose/formaldehyde gel. The mRNA was then transferred to nitrocellulose [18], baked for 2 h and hybridized with a 1.2-kb human EPO cDNA probe that had been labelled with α^{32}-P-dCTP. The nitrocellulose was then washed and autoradiographed. To normalize any variation in amounts of mRNA, the nitrocellulose was reprobed with a control α-Tubulin cDNA probe as described above. The autoradiographs were analyzed by scanning densitometry and the results expressed as intensity of EPO/intensity of Tubulin.

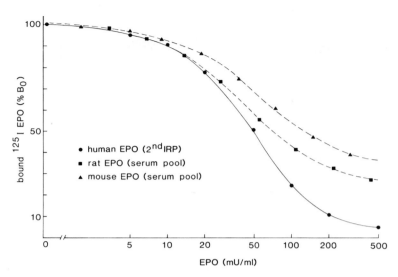

Fig. 1. Standard curves of the EPO RIA, demonstrating cross-reactivity of rat and mouse EPO with the antiserum derived against human recombinant EPO. The total amount of antibody-precipitable ^{125}I EPO in the absence of unlabelled EPO (B_0) was on average 45% of the radioactivity added.

Factors Affecting Circulating EPO Levels

Circulating EPO levels were found to be decreased or increased under a variety of conditions. Many of these are characterized by *alterations of oxygen delivery* to tissues. Anemia, caused by bleeding or a hypofunctional bone marrow, is the most powerful stimulus for a rise of serum EPO [19], with an exponential relation between EPO levels and the fall of hematocrit [13]. Inhalation of carbon monoxide, which causes a functional reduction of the oxygen transport capacity of the blood, is also associated with a large increase in serum EPO concentration [20, 21]. Furthermore, the oxygen affinity of hemoglobin affects blood levels of EPO in that an increase of oxygen affinity leads to a rise in the EPO levels [22]. Another important stimulus for increased EPO production is a fall of the arterial oxygen tension caused by either cardiopulmonary disorders or by a decrease of the oxygen tension in the inspiratory gas. Conversely, an increase in red cell mass as in polycythemia vera is associated with low EPO levels [23, 24]. In addition to changes in oxygen delivery, *metabolic factors* also influence EPO production. Hypophysectomy [25, 26] and starvation [13] are accompanied by decreased EPO titers whilst stimulation of metabolism by thyroid hormone [27] increases EPO concentrations. Finally, circulating EPO levels can also be enhanced by the administration of *cobalt* [28]. While this stimulation by cobalt does not seem to reflect a general regulatory principle (see below), all the other observations can be summarized in that states of reduced oxygen supply and states of increased oxygen demand are accompanied by increased levels of circulating EPO, whilst suppressed levels of EPO are typical for conditions with increased oxygen supply or reduced oxygen demand. The physiological role of EPO therefore seems to be the adjustment of red cell production to the oxygen demand of the tissues.

Renal Oxygen Sensor

No evidence exists that the clearance rate of EPO is subject to a physiological regulation. We may infer therefore that the plasma concentration of EPO directly reflects the renal secretion rate, which is apparently under the control of an *oxygen sensor* that is sensitive to the ratio of oxygen supply to oxygen demand. A priori, it is not clear whether this oxygen sensor is located in the kidney and it was obvious to look for a role of the classical chemoreceptors in the regulation of EPO production. However, neither carotid body function nor any other neural input into the kidney seems to be necessary for the enhancement of EPO synthesis in response to hypoxia [29, 30]. On the other hand, selective reduction of renal blood flow is able to elicit an increase of EPO formation [31, 33]. Also the isolated perfused kidney releases more EPO upon lowering the oxygen tension in the perfusate [34, 35] and in addition even renal tissue cultures produce more EPO after exposure to lower oxygen tensions [36, 37a]. It is likely therefore that the oxygen sensor controlling EPO synthesis is indeed located in the kidney itself.

The localization of this oxygen sensor within the kidney, however, is yet unknown. From it's function, namely the determination of an oxygen supply to demand ratio, the sensor should be related to structures with high energy demand and in consequence high oxygen consumption. Oxygen consumption of the kidney is primarily determined by the rate of tubular sodium reabsorption [38]. To narrow down the possible localizations of the oxygen sensor, we examined the effect of site-specific inhibition of sodium reabsorption in different parts of the nephron on EPO production. For that

Table I. Effect of diuretics on hypoxia-induced EPO production

	Acetazol-amide		Furosemide		Thiazide		Amiloride	
Site of action	proximal tubule		loop of Henle		distal tubule		collecting duct	
Normal Na$^+$ reabsorption at respective segment, % of filtered load	60		30		8		1	
Na$^+$ excretion under diuretic therapy, % of filtered load	3		23		5		5	
	C	T	C	T	C	T	C	T
Serum EPO in response to 3 h 8% O$_2$, mU/ml n	309 ±17 20	348 ±26 15	265 ±18 28	317 ±23 30	314 ±60 5	300 ±27 5	237 ±33 15	233 ±23 15
Serum EPO in response to 3 h 0.1% CO, mU/ml n	727 ±92 5	586 ±84 5	727 ±92 5	702 ±92 5	625 ±36 5	532 ±50 5	625 ±36 5	643 ±40 5

Application of diuretic drugs did not lead to a significant reduction of EPO response. However, the effect of acetazolamide on proximal tubule sodium absorption is likely to be too small to significantly reduce oxygen consumption of this segment. Na excretion under diuretics is expressed in relation to Na excretion of control animals (46 µmol/5 animals within 3 h), which was assumed to be 1% of filtered load. C = Control; T = treated.

purpose, diuretic drugs were administered to mice prior to hypoxic exposure. The results are documented in table I and they make clear that effective inhibition of sodium reabsorption in the collecting duct, distal tubule, macula densa region and loop of Henle does not reduce the degree of hypoxia as perceived by the oxygen sensor. In our experiments we were, however, not able to sufficiently inhibit proximal tubular sodium absorption. By exclusion we infer that if the oxygen sensor is at all related to tubular function it should be at the proximal tubular site. Apart from the cellular localization of the oxygen-sensing mechanism, the cell type *producing* EPO has also not yet been identified unequivocally. Since EPO is not stored in the cells, they cannot be identified by means of immunohistochemistry, but can only be defined by their ability to produce mRNA for EPO. Recent and

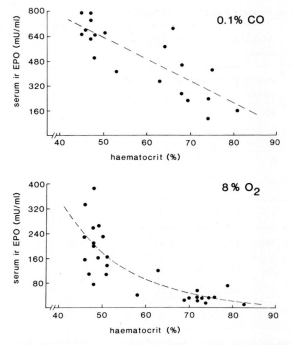

Fig. 2. Hypoxia-induced EPO response. Inverse correlation between hematocrit and serum EPO levels in response to (i) carbon monoxide inhalation for 3 h and (ii) hypoxic hypoxia for 3 h. The figure includes normal animals (Hct $\leq 53\%$) and animals studied 4 or 12 days after a previous exposure to normobaric hypoxia for 15 days (Hct 74.8 ± 1.5 and $67.7 \pm 1.4\%$; $\bar{x} \pm SEM$, n = 12 and 11, respectively).

strong evidence indicates that the mRNA for EPO is present in renal cortical cells in close proximity to the proximal tubule [see 37b]. This localization of the EPO-producing cells would well fit with the concept that the proximal tubule takes part in the process of oxygen sensing.

Before discussing the possibilities how the proximal tubule could be involved in this sensing process, we should look at the parameter that is measured by the oxygen sensor. From the above mentioned it is obvious that the oxygen sensor is sensitive to (i) conditions that affect arterial pO_2 and consequently also venous pO_2 (e. g. hypoxic hypoxia) and (ii) conditions in which arterial pO_2 is normal and only venous pO_2 is changed due to altered oxygen transport capacity (e. g. anemia). The question therefore arises whether the oxygen sensor is, apart from sensing postcapillary (venous) pO_2 as in condition (ii), also able to measure precapillary (arterial) pO_2. Figure 2 shows however that the extent of stimulation of EPO production by both arterial hypoxia and functional anemia (carbon monoxide inhalation) is inversely related to the oxygen transport capacity of the blood. This indicates that in both conditions the postcapillary rather than the precapillary pO_2 is being sensed.

Presently we do not know whether the EPO-producing cell itself behaves functionally as an oxygen sensor. If this were the case, the function of the proximal tubular cells might be that of a regulated sink for oxygen because their own oxygen consumption would bring the pO_2 around the EPO-producing cells to varying venous values. If, on the other hand, the EPO-producing cells themselves are not acting as an oxygen sensor, it would be likely that the proximal tubular cells generate a biochemical signal upon hypoxia that triggers EPO production in adjacent cells.

Cellular Regulation of EPO Production

It is well established that the kidneys contain no stores for EPO [39, 40]. Moreover, a comparison of the nucleotide sequence of the mRNA for EPO and the amino acid sequence of the molecule reveals that EPO is not synthesized as an activatable precursor [5, 6]. Additional evidence indicates that EPO is not sequestered into specific secretory granules on its pathway from synthesis to secretion [R. Taugner, pers. commun.]. One may infer therefore that the secretion of EPO is regulated by the rate of synthesis. This in turn is necessarily determined by the cellular content of EPO mRNA and may in addition be modulated by changes of the translation rate. To evaluate whether changes of the translation rate play a significant role, we compared the EPO mRNA content of rat kidneys during hypoxia with serum EPO levels (fig. 3). The Northern blot technique used is not sensitive enough to detect the low mRNA levels present in normoxic animals and we could also not detect EPO mRNA in response to a mild hypoxic stimulus (13.5% O_2), though serum EPO did already increase significantly (data not shown). However, with a higher degree of hypoxia (10.5% O_2) we observed a linear increase of EPO mRNA that paralleled the increase of serum EPO. This indicates that at least under the present experimental conditions the production of EPO is directly regulated by changes of EPO mRNA content.

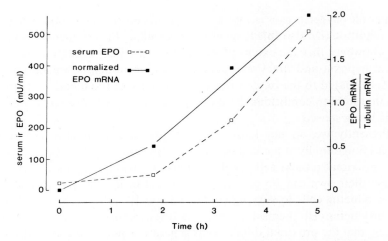

Fig. 3. The increase of serum EPO levels in rats during hypoxia is paralleled by an increase of renal EPO mRNA. EPO mRNA content was quantitated by analyzing Northern blot autoradiographs with scanning densitometry and the respective intensity expressed in relation to the intensity resulting after hybridization of the same blot with an α-Tubulin probe. Hypoxia corresponded to 10.5% O_2.

Before discussing the mechanisms that might lead to an activation of the EPO gene, we should consider the time lapse between the onset of the hypoxic stimulus and the first detectable rise of EPO in the blood. Compatible with previous observations [41, 42], we found that independent of the kind of hypoxic stimulus, the degree of hypoxia and the species studied (man, rat, mouse), the delay between onset of the stimulus and rise of serum EPO is between 1 and 1.5 h (fig. 4). This time span includes the following partial steps: (i) washout of the oxygen stores in the body; (ii) signal recognition and transduction at the oxygen sensor; (iii) transcription of the EPO gene and translation of EPO mRNA, and (iv) translocation of EPO and equilibration of the distribution space. In order to get an idea about the time required for the activation of the oxygen sensor, we exposed mice to a hypoxic stimulus for 5, 15 or 30 min – time periods after which serum EPO has not yet risen (fig. 4) – and allowed another 3 h in normoxic atmosphere after termination of the hypoxic stimulus, before determining serum EPO levels. Once the oxygen sensor was activated during the short hypoxic exposures, production of EPO could then proceed during this following time period. EPO levels did not change after 5 and 15 min of hypoxia but

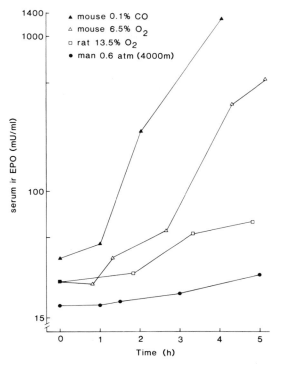

Fig. 4. Time-dependent increase of serum EPO levels in man, rat and mouse in response to different hypoxic stimuli.

increased significantly after 30 min (34.1 ± 4.9 vs. 20.9 ± 2.7 mU/ml, p<0.001), thus indicating that the time required for stimulation of the oxygen sensor is maximally 30 min. So far, we do not know whether the onset of gene transcription is already included in this period; however, 60 min after the onset of hypoxia a clear increase in EPO mRNA has been demonstrated [43]. Thus at least 30 min seem to be neessary for synthesis, cellular export and distribution of EPO.

In the following we will discuss the mechanism that might link a local fall of pO_2 to an enhanced transcription of the EPO gene. The knowledge about this process is still very fragmentary, because the cell culture models available [36, 37, 44, 45] produce much smaller amounts of EPO than the intact kidney and are not proven to be derived from cells that produce EPO in vivo. Therefore some findings derived from in vitro studies that are currently included in concepts of cellular regulation of EPO production await further review once the question of the cellular location is solved.

It seems reasonable to assume that the pO_2 does not directly regulate gene transcription, which in turn necessitates a signal transduction with the consecutive generation of metabolic messenger molecules. For instance, a change in pO_2 could be indicated by changing the turnover rate of oxygen-dependent enyzmes, like oxidases. The pO_2 could also be sensed by the energy metabolism, in particular by the respiratory chain producing ATP. We have recently provided evidence that an instantaneous increase of energy consumption in renal tubular cells in vitro, brought about by stimulation of the NaCl transport, leads to an increase of the ADP/ATP ratio at the plasma membrane where the Na/K ATPase is located [46]. As a result of this local fall of the ATP concentration, reacylation of arachidonic acid was attenuated leading to an enhanced release of prostaglandins. Furthermore, the key enzymes of glycolysis were stimulated under this condition, leading to an enhanced release of lactate. Thus in a condition of mismatch between oxygen supply and oxygen demand, two different substances, prostaglandin and lactate, are being released that could act as messenger molecules. And in fact, among the biochemical parameters that might link a fall of pO_2 with enhanced transcription of the EPO gene, *prostaglandins* are being seriously considered as candidates. This is based on the findings that (i) several tissues including the kidney release more prostaglandins upon hypoxia [47, 48], (ii) prostaglandins are able to enhance EPO release from the kidney [49, 50] and also in cell culture models [51], and (iii) inhibition of prostaglandin formation inhibits renal EPO formation in vivo in response to hypoxia [21, 52, 53].

How could prostaglandins then affect EPO gene transcription? A second messenger signal that could be involved in signal transmission is *cyclic AMP,* because it has been found that activators of the adenylate cyclase, including prostaglandins, stimulate EPO formation in vivo and in vitro [44, 51, 54]. A further well-established, but nevertheless mysterious stimulator of EPO production is *cobalt.* It has been demonstrated that cobalt treatment causes a significant rise in renal EPO mRNA [10, 43]. As shown in figure 5, the stimulatory effect of cobalt is not blunted by increasing the oxygen transport capacity of the blood, suggesting that cobalt acts at a site distal of the oxygen-sensing mechanism. In contrast to hypoxia-stimulated EPO formation, cobalt-stimulated EPO formation is not attenuated by prostaglandin synthesis inhibition [21], which further supports the notion that cobalt has no effect on the first steps of the oxygen-sensing mechanism. In all

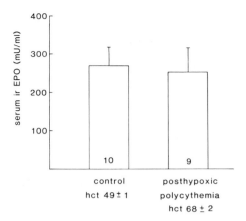

Fig. 5. Cobalt-induced EPO response. Serum EPO levels 12 h after subcutaneous administration of cobalt chloride in normal and polycythemic mice that were previously exposed to a 15-day period of normobaric hypoxia ($\bar{x} \pm$ SEM).

tissues so far investigated, cobalt is known as an inhibitor of all types of calcium channels [e. g. 55]. One may speculate therefore that cobalt exerts its effect by blocking the calcium influx into EPO-producing cells. In fact, the calcium entry blockers verapamil and diltiazem as well as a low calcium medium have been demonstrated to enhance EPO secretion in a renal carcinoma cell culture system [45]. These date are supported by in vivo studies, in which it was demonstrated that verapamil enhances the effect of hypoxia on EPO production [56, and own data not shown]. It might be of interest in this context that a rise of the cAMP concentration leads to a fall in the intracellular calcium concentration in several tissues by inhibiting calcium entry across the cell membrane. These results would raise the possibility that the EPO gene is normally under the inhibitory control of a calcium-calmodulin-dependent process. Lowering the intracellular calcium concentration by physiological or pharmacological (verapamil, cobalt) means would then be a stimulatory signal for EPO production.

Acknowledgements

We are indebted to Dr. P. Hirth, Boehringer Mannheim GmbH, for the generous gift of anti-EPO antiserum and to Dr. C. B. Shoemaker, Genetics Institute, for providing us with the cDNA probe of the human EPO gene. The authors' work was supported by the

Swiss National Science Foundation (grants 3.023–0.84), the Roche Research Foundation and the Hartmann Müller Stiftung für medizinische Forschung. K.-U. E. acknowledges a fellowship from the Deutsche Forschungsgemeinschaft.

References

1   Carnot, P.; Deflandre, C.: Sur l'activité hémopoiétique des différents organes au cours de la régénération d sang. C.r. hebd. Séanc. Acad. Sci., Paris *143:* 432–435 (1906).

2   Peschle, C.; Condorelli, M.: Biogenesis of erythropoietin: evidence for pro-erythropoietin in a subcellular fraction of the kidney. Science *190:* 910–912 (1975).

3   Gordon, A. S.; Cooper, G. W.; Zanjani, E. D.: The kidney and erythropoiesis. Semin. Hematol. *4:* 337–358 (1967).

4   Miyake, T.; Kung, C. K. H.; Goldwasser, E.: Purification of human erythropoietin. J. biol. Chem. *252:* 5558–5564 (1977).

5   Lai, P.-H.; Everett, R.; Wang, F.-F.; Arakawa, T.; Goldwasser, E.: Structural characterization of human erythropoietin. J. biol. Chem. *261:* 3116–3121 (1986).

6   McDonald, J. D.; Lin, F.-K.; Goldwasser, E.: Cloning, sequencing and evolutionary analysis of the mouse erythropoietin gene. Mol. cell. Biol. *6:* 842–848 (1986).

7   Jacobs, K.; Shoemaker, C.; Rudersdorf, R.; Neill, S. D.; Kaufman, R. J.; Mufson, A.; Seehra, J.; Jones, S. S.; Hewick, R.; Fritsch, E. F.; Kawakita, M.; Shimizu, T.; Miyake, T.: Isolation and characterization of genomic and cDNA clones of human erythropoietin. Nature, Lond. *313:* 806–810 (1985).

8   Lin, F.-K.; Suggs, S.; Lin, C.-H.; Browne, J. K.; Smalling, R.; Egrie, J. C.; Chen, K. K.; Fox, G. M.; Martin, F.; Stabinski, Z.; Badrawi, M.; Lai, P.-H.; Goldwasser, E.: Cloning and expression of the human erythropoietin gene. Proc. natn. Acad. Sci. USA *82:* 7580–7584 (1985).

9   Bondurant, M. C:; Koury, M. J.: Anemia induces accumulation of erythropoietin mRNA in the kidney and liver. Mol. cell. Biol. *6:* 2731–2733 (1986).

10 Beru, N.; McDonald, J.; Lacombe, C.; Goldwasser, E.: Expression of the erythropoietin gene. Mol. cell. Biol. *6:* 2571–2575 (1986).

11 Zanjani, E. D.; Peterson, E. N.; Gordon, A. S.; Wasserman, L. R.: Erythropoietin production in the fetus: role of the kidney and maternal anemia. J. Lab. clin. Med. *83:* 281–287 (1974).

12 Jacobson, L. O.; Goldwasser, E.; Fried, W.; Plzak, L. F.: The role of the kidney in erythropoiesis. Nature, Lond. *179:* 633–634 (1957).

13 Jelkmann, W.: Renal erythropoietin: properties and production. Rev. Physiol. Biochem. Pharmacol. *104:* 140–215 (1986).

14 Eckardt, K.-U.; Kurtz, A.; Hirth, P.; Scigalla, P.; Wieczorek, L.; Bauer, C.: Evaluation of the stability of human erythropoietin in samples for radioimmunoassay. Klin. Wschr. (in press).

15 Cotes, P. M.; Bangham, D. R.: Bioassay for erythropoietin in mice made polycythemic by exposure to air at a reduced pressure. Nature, Lond. *191:* 1065–1067 (1961).

16 Chirgwin, J.: Przybyla, A. E.; MacDonald, R. J.; Rutter, W. J.: Isolation of biologi-

cally active ribonucleic acid from sources enriched in ribonuclease. Biochemistry *18:* 5294–5299 (1977).

17 Aviv, H.; Leder, P.: Purification of biologically active globin messenger RNA by chromatography on oligothymidylic acid-cellulose. Proc. natn. Acad. Sci. USA *69:* 1408–1412 (1972).

18 Thomas, P. S.: Hybridization of denatured RNA and small DNA fragments transferred to nitrocellulose. Proc. natn. Acad. Sci. USA *77:* 5201–5205 (1980).

19 Erslev, A. J.; Caro, J.; Miller, O.; Silver, R.: Plasma erythropoietin in health and disease. Ann. clin. Lab. Sci. *10:* 250–257 (1980).

20 Syvertsen, G. R.; Harris, J. A.: Erythropoietin production in dogs exposed to high altitude and carbon monoxide. Am. J. Physiol. *225:* 293–299 (1973).

21 Jelkmann, W.; Kurtz, A.; Seidl, J.; Bauer, C.: Mechanisms of the renal glomerular erythropoietin production; in Grote, Witzleb, Atemgaswechsel und O_2-Versorgung der Organe, pp. 130–137 (Akademie der Wissenschaften und der Literatur, Mainz 1984).

22 Lechermann, B.; Jelkmann, W.: Erythropoietin production in normoxic and hypoxic rats with increased blood O_2 affinity. Resp. Physiol. *60:* 1–8 (1985).

23 Erslev, A. J.; Caro, J.; Kansu, E.; Miller, O.; Cobbs, E.: Plasma erythropoietin in polycyctemia. Am. J. Med. *66:* 243–247 (1979).

24 Garcia, J. F.; Ebbe, S. N.; Hollander, L.; Cutting, H. O.; Miller, M. E.; Cronkite, E. P.: Radioimmunoassay of erythropoietin: circulating levels in normal and poylcythemic human beings. J. Lab. clin. Med. *99:* 624–635 (1982).

25 Peschle, C.; Rappaport, I. A.; Magli, M. C.; Marone, G.; Lettieri, F.; Cillo, C.; Gordon, A. S.: Role of the hypophysis in erythropoietin production during hypoxia. Blood *51:* 1117–1124 (1978).

26 Halvorsen, S.; Roh, B. L.; Fisher, J. W.: Erythropoietin production in nephrectomized and hypophysectomized animals. Am. J. Physiol. *215:* 349–352 (1968).

27 Peschle, C.; Zanjani, E. D.; Gidari, A. S.; McLaurin, W. D.; Gordon, A. S.: Mechanism of thyroxine action on erythropoiesis. Endocrinology *89:* 609–612 (1971).

28 Goldwasser, E.; Jacobson, L. O.; Fried, W.; Plzak, L. F.: Studies on erythropoiesis. V. The effect of cobalt on the production of erythropoietin. Blood *13:* 55–60 (1958).

29 Hansen, A. J.: Fogh, J.; Møllgard, K.; Sørensen, S. C.: Evidence against EPO production by the carotid body. Resp. Physiol. *18:* 101–106 (1973).

30 Beynon, G.: The influence of the autonomic nervous system in the control of erythropoietin secretion in the hypoxic rat. J. Physiol. *266:* 347–360 (1977).

31 Takaku, F.; Hirashima, K.; Nakao, K.: Studies on the mechanism of erythropoietin production. I. Effect of unilateral constriction of the renal artery. J. Lab. clin. Med. *59:* 815–820 (1962).

32 Hansen, P.: Polycythemia produced by constriction of the renal artery in a rabbit. Acta pathol. microbiol. immunol. scand. *60:* 465–472 (1964).

33 Fisher, J. W.; Samuels. A. I.: Relationship between renal blood flow and erythropoietin production in dogs. Proc. Soc. exp. biol. Med. *125:* 482–485 (1967).

34 Kuratowska, Z.; Lewartowski, B.; Michalak, E.: Studies on the production of erythropoietin by isolated perfused organs. Blood *18:* 527–534 (1961).

35 Fisher, J. W.; Langston, J. W.: Effects of testosterone, cobalt and hypoxia on erythropoietin production in the isolated perfused dog kidney. Ann. N.Y. Acad. Sci. *149:* 75–87 (1968).

36   Kurtz, A.; Jelkmann, W.; Sinowatz, F.; Bauer, C.: Renal mesangial cell cultures as a model for study of erythropoietin production. Proc. natn. Acad. Sci. USA 80: 4008–4011 (1983).

37a Caro, J. Hickey, J.; Erslev, A.: Erythropoietin production by an established kidney proximal tubule cell line (LLCPK$_1$). Exp. Hematol. 12: 357 (1984).

37b Lacombe, C.; Da Silva, J. L.; Bruneval, P.; Camilleri, J. P.; Bariety, J.; Tambourin, P.; Varet, B.: Identification of tissues and cells producing erythropoietin in the anemic mouse. Contr. Nephrol., vol. 66, pp. 17–24 (Karger, Basel 1988).

38   Deetjen, P.; Kramer, K.: Die Abhängigkeit des O$_2$-Verbrauchs der Niere von der Na$^+$ Rückresorption. Pflügers Arch. 273: 636–650 (1961).

39   Sherwood, J. B.; Goldwasser, E.: Extraction of erythropoietin from normal kidneys. Endocrinology 103: 866–870 (1978).

40   Jelkmann, W.; Bauer, C.: Demonstration of high levels of erythropoietin in rat kidneys following hypoxic hypoxia. Pflügers Arch. 393: 34–39 (1981).

41   Schooley, J. C.; Mahlmann, L. J.: Evidence for the de novo synthesis of erythropoietin in hypoxic rats. Blood 40: 662–670 (1972).

42   Clemons, G. C.; DeManincor, D.; Fitzsimmons, S. L.; Garcia, J. F.: Immunoreactive erythropoietin studies in hypoxic rats and the role of the salivary glands. Exp. Hematol. 15: 18–23 (1987).

43   Schuster, S. J.; Wilson, J. H.; Erslev, A. J.; Caro, J.: Physiologic regulation and tissue localization of renal erythropoietin messenger RNA. Blood 70: 316–318 (1987).

44   Sherwood, J. B:; Burns, E. R.; Shouval, D.: Stimulation by cAMP of erythropoietin secretion by an established human renal carcinoma cell line. Blood 69: 1053–1057 (1987).

45   Nagakura, K.; Fisher, J. W.: Low levels of calcium increase erythropoietin (Ep) secretion by human renal carcinoma cells in culture. Fed. Proc. 45: 655 (1986).

46   Kurtz, A.; Pfeilschifter, J.; Malmström, K.; Woodson, R. D.; Bauer, C.: Mechanism of NaCl transport-stimulated prostaglandin formation in MDCK cells. Am. J. Physiol. 252: C307–C314 (1987).

47   Gross, D. M.; Mujovic, V. M.; Jubiz, W.; Fisher, J. W.: Enhanced erythropoietin and prostaglandin E production in the dog following renal artery constriction. Proc. Soc. exp. Biol. Med. 151: 498–501 (1976).

48   Walker, B. R.: Diuretic response to acute hypoxia in the conscious dog. Am. J. Physiol. 243: F440–F446 (1982).

49   Foley, J. W.; Gross, D. M.; Nelson, P. K.; Fisher, J. W.: The effects of arachidonic acid on erythropoietin production in exhypoxic polycythemic mice and the isolated perfused canine kidney. J. Pharmac. exp. Ther. 207: 402–409 (1978).

50   Gross, D. M.; Fisher, J. W.; Erythropoietic effects of PGE$_2$ and two-endoperoxide analogs. Experientia 36: 458–459 (1980).

51   Kurtz, A.; Jelkmann, W.; Pfeilschifter, J.; Bauer, C.: Role of prostaglandins in hypoxia-stimulated erythopoietin production. Am. J. Physiol. 249: C3–C8 (1985).

52   Mujovic, V. M.; Fisher, J. W.: The role of prostaglandins in the production of erythropoietin (ESF) by the kidney. II. Effects of indomethacin on erythropoietin production following hypoxia in dogs. Life Sci. 16: 463–473 (1975).

53   Fisher, J. W.: Prostaglandins and kidney erythropoietin production. Nephron 25: 53–56 (1980).

54   Rodgers, G. M.; Fisher, J. W.; George, J. W.: The role of adenosine 3', 5',-mono-

phosphate in the control of erythropoietin production. Am. J. Med. *58:* 31–38 (1975).

55 Kohlhardt, M.; Bauer, B.; Krause, H.; Fleckenstein, A.: Selective inhibition of the transmembrane Ca conductivity of mammalian myocardial fibers by Ni, Co and Mn ions. Pflügers Arch. *388:* 115–123 (1973).
56 McGonigle, R. J. S.; Brookins, J.; Pegram, B. L.; Fisher, J. W.: Enhanced erythropoietin production by calcium entry blockers in rats exposed to hypoxia. J. Pharmac. exp. Ther. *241:* 428–432 (1987).

Dr. Armin Kurtz, Physiologisches Institut, Universität Zürich, Winterthurerstrasse 190, CH-8057 Zürich (Switzerland)

Discussion

Müller-Wiefel: Dr. Kurtz, could you briefly comment on the hypothesis of β_2-adrenergic stimulation of EPO synthesis?

Kurtz: Data were obtained, to my knowledge, with the model of the isolated perfused kidney – with the programmed kidney – and I know of no clear evidence that β_2-adrenergic agonists stimulate EPO formation in vivo. But if you could provide some direct information that they stimulate EPO formation in vivo then I would accept this, of course.

Müller-Wiefel: I would agree with your opinion from the clinical point of view because we have never seen a negative effect on erythropoiesis by β-blocking agents.

Koch: On your last slide you showed that in addition to the capillary endothelium, you also suspect or discussed the marcophage as a source of EPO production. What is the present status of this concept?

Kurtz: I would like to give an answer, but I think it is the topic of Dr. Varet to present the results and discuss the cell type.

Pfäffl: Do we have experimental evidence that clamping of the renal artery increases the EPO output?

Kurtz: Yes, there is a direct experimental evidence. However, the rise of EPO following clamping the renal artery is relatively small. So, if I remember correctly, lowering the renal blood flow to about 20% increases EPO values from 20 mU/ml to 100 or 150. It is in no case the rise that is observed during hypoxia or anemia.

Bauer: Perhaps, Dr. Pfäffl, I might add that there are several case reports in which it was shown that, after kidney transplantation, one gets a huge increase in EPO and red cell mass, and if you do renal angiography you will find vascular abnormalities. If you correct this redistribution of intrarenal blood flow, then the EPO goes back. So you really don't need a massive reduction of renal blood flow, but rather an intrarenal looping of blood flow. There are rather nicely documented cases on this.

Koch: Just a comment to Dr. Pfäffl's question. Isn't this really what you expect when you reduce the blood flow of the kidney. You have less filtration and less sodium transport and less oxygen consumption. So, you don't stimulate the system as much as you would if you had hypoxemia.

Kurtz: In our opinion this is the reason why the increase of EPO is relatively small in comparison with hypoxia, because by reducing perfusion one also decreases the energy consumption of the kidney.

Caro: Do you have any further comments about your experiments with blockade of sodium reabsorption and its inability to show any effect on EPO production?

Kurtz: No, so far we have no positive result. We can effectively block the sodium reabsorption in the distal tubule, in the collecting duct and in the loop of Henle and these manipulations do not at all affect EPO production. I think we were not able to effectively block proximal tubular sodium reabsorption.

Nattermann: Is there an interrelation between the EPO production and the renin production? So when we have high EPO levels we also have high renin levels?

Kurtz: Is that really true that in every case there is direct correlation? I am not sure that each state of high EPO is parallelled by high renin. And, in particular, renin synthesis and its regulation is very poorly understood. Renin is stored in granules and alterations in the blood plasma levels are due to secretion of renin and the blood levels of renin are controlled by the exocytotic process. In the case of EPO, the blood levels are controlled by de novo synthesis and by gene transcription. I therefore think it is very difficult to compare renin synthesis and EPO synthesis by comparing the blood levels of both molecules. From my experience it is not right to say that every state of high EPO is accompanied by high renin.

Winearls (London): There are reports that captopril makes a difference to EPO production. Do you know whether that is due to an effect on the blood flow?

Kurtz: Yes, I heard about it, but we have no experience at the moment and no explanation on the phenomenon that inhibitors of the converting enzyme are associated with decreased levels of EPO.

Grützmacher: May I confirm these data. We measured after orally ingested captopril EPO as well as renin and you can very clearly demonstrate a selective increase of renin at the presence of a constant EPO level.

Contr. Nephrol., vol. 66, pp. 17–24 (Karger, Basel 1988)

Identification of Tissues and Cells Producing Erythropoietin in the Anemic Mouse

Catherine Lacombe[a], *Jean-Louis Da Silva*[b], *Patrick Bruneval*[b], *Jean-Pierre Camilleri*[b], *Jean Bariety*[b], *Pierre Tambourin*[a], *Bruno Varet*[a]

[a]INSERM U.152, Hôpital Cochin, and [b]INSERM U.28, Hôpital Boussais, Paris, France

Erythropoietin (EPO) is the glycoprotein growth factor which controls red blood cell production in mammals. EPO synthesis is regulated via feedback mechanisms involving tissue oxygen tension. Until recently, physiological studies of EPO production were mostly based upon indirect evidence. Since the work of Jacobson et al. [1], the central role of the kidney was a well-recognized fact [for review, see 2]. Other sites of EPO production nevertheless exist, since some degree of hypoxia-regulated erythropoiesis persists in the majority of anephric mammals. The liver was the only extrarenal organ that has been proved to release EPO into the blood. Other organs such as the salivary glands, spleen, and bone marrow have been implicated. The identity of the cells responsible for EPO production was still a greater matter of controversy. A glomerular origin has been suggested based on immunohistochemical studies [3, 4] and on studies on EPO production by in vitro cultures of glomerular [5] and mesangial [6] cells. Proximal tubular cells have also been considered as excellent candidates [7]. Macrophages, at least in culture, have also been reported to produce EPO [8].

The recent molecular cloning of the EPO gene has provided a powerful tool to further analyze EPO biosynthesis [9–12]. Using the murine EPO gene as a probe, a rapid EPO mRNA accumulation has been demonstrated in the kidney of adult rodents under hypoxic conditions [13, 14]. Very recently, Schuster et al. [15] have shown that EPO mRNA was not synthesized by the glomerular but by the tubular fraction of the hypoxic kidney. We used the murine EPO gene probe to localize EPO mRNA synthesis in mice made deeply anemic to increase their production of EPO.

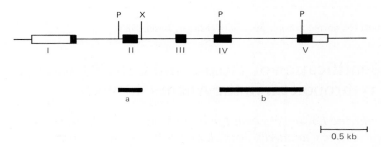

Fig. 1. Schematic map of the mouse EPO gene and of the two DNA probes used. Exons are indicated by Roman numerals. P = *Pst*I; X = *Xho*II.

Materials and Methods

Induction of EPO Production. Mice were made profoundly anemic by a 6-Gy irradiation followed 24 h later by an intraperitoneal injection of phenylhydrazine (60 mg/kg b.w.). Nine to 10 days later, they were bled for serum EPO titration and their organs removed. The organs were half frozen in liquid nitrogen for subsequent in situ hybridization, and the second half processed for poly-(A)$^+$ RNA isolation. The EPO level in the plasma of these anemic mice was shown to be between 6 and 10 IU/ml of serum.

EPO Probes. Two genomic DNA probes were used (fig. 1). Probe a was a 243-bp *Pst*I-*Xho*II restriction fragment encompassing the second exon of the mouse EPO gene which was inserted at the *Pst*I and *Bam*HI sites of a pUC18 vector. A 265-bp EPO insert/pUC18 *Pst*I-*Eco* RI-purified fragment was derived from this construct. Probe b was a 1-kb *Pst*I-*Pst*I EPO genomic fragment containing part of exon IV and part of exon V.

Northern Blot Analysis. RNAs were extracted from organs by the hot phenol procedure [16]. Total RNAs were purified by oligo-(dT) affinity chromatography to obtain poly-(A)$^+$ RNA-enriched preparations. After glyoxal denaturation and transfer to Gene Screen Plus membranes, the RNAs were hybridized with ^{32}P-labeled probe b (specific activity 2.10^8 cpm/µg of DNA).

In situ Hybridization. The procedure used for in situ hybridization has been previously described [17].

Immunohistochemical Techniques. Willebrand factor was checked with an anti-human Willebrand factor polyclonal rabbit antibody (Dakopatts, Copenhagen, Denmark) using the indirect immunofluorescence technique. The monoclonal anti-F4/80 antibody, which recognizes a membrane antigen specific for murine monocytes-macrophages [18] (kindly provided by G. Milon, Institut Pasteur, Paris), was revealed using the peroxidase-antiperoxidase technique.

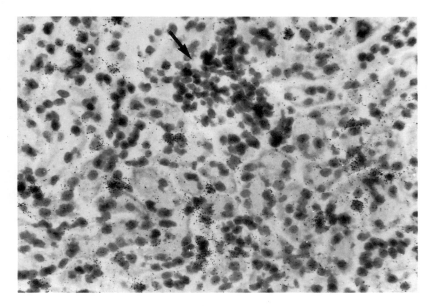

Fig. 2. In situ hybridization with the ^{35}S-labeled EPO genomic probe on the renal cortex of an anemic mouse. The arrow indicates the glomerulus. Numerous silver grains labeled most peritubular cells, whereas the glomerular cells and the tubular epithelial cells remained negative ×315.

Results and Discussion

EPO mRNA Expression in Organs of Hypoxic Mice

On Northern blot hybridized with EPO probe, a 1.8-kb band was observed in the poly-(A$^+$) RNAs extracted from the kidney and the liver of anemic mice. This size is identical to the murine EPO RNA previously described [13, 14]. The ratio of liver/kidney per microgram of mRNA can be estimated to be about ¼. Other organs (brain, salivary glands, testis) were all negative even after a longer exposure of the film (10 days). These data confirm previous results of other groups [13–15] showing that the liver and the kidney are the only organs which produce significant amount of EPO in the hypoxic adult mouse. The previous suggestions that other organs contained biologically reactive or immunoreactive EPO can be explained either by a storage of the protein in these organs, or the lack of specificity of the techniques used to measure EPO.

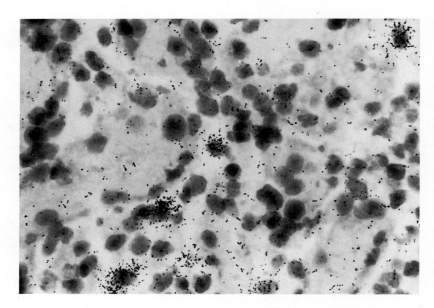

Fig. 3. Higher magnification of the renal cortex of an anemic mouse showing the extratubular location of the labeled cells. ×610.

Identification of Cells Which Produce EPO [19]

On the sections of hypoxic kidneys hybridized with the EPO probe, clusters of silver grains were observed on cells located in the cortex and the outer medulla. Glomerular and tubular epithelial cells were negative as well as cells of arteries, arterioles and veins (fig. 2). At higher magnification (fig. 3), all the positive cells appeared to be in a peritubular location. Statistical analysis confirmed that the number of grains was higher on peritubular cells than on other cells of the cortex and the outer medulla. The number of labeled peritubular cells seemed to be higher in the cortex than in the outer medulla but the difference was significant only in 2/4 kidneys studied [20].

No significant labeling was observed in the inner medulla. Kidney sections from anemic mice either treated with RNase before hybridization or hybridized with a ^{35}S-labeled pUC18 vector without the EPO insert were negative. On the liver cells from hypoxic animals, no obvious specific labeling was observed.

The location and the morphology of the EPO-producing cells suggest that they are endothelial capillary cells [21]. In the human kidney, peritubular cells are known to be genuine endothelial cells containing Willebrand factor [22]. Our immunofluorescence data using Willebrand factor antibody show that the same is true in the murine kidney [19]. Macrophages have also been described to produce EPO in culture [8]. However, we find that macrophages are not the EPO-producing cells in the hypoxic kidney, since in the area where EPO cells were located, no staining with the anti-F4/80 antibody was observed [19].

To demonstrate that peritubular cells which produce EPO under hypoxia are genuine endothelial cells, double labelling with the EPO probe and an anti-Willebrand factor antibody must be performed. Whatever the precise lineage of these peritubular cells, it is very likely that the oxygen-sensitive cells are the tubular cells and not the EPO-producing cells. This suggests that a (soluble?) factor is produced by tubular cells to stimulate EPO production in their neighborhood.

References

1   Jacobson, L. O.; Goldwasser, E.; Fried, W.; Plzak, L.: Role of the kidney in erythro-poiesis. Nature, Lond. *179:* 633–634 (1957).
2   Jelkmann, W.: Renal erythropoietin: Properties and Production. Rev. Physiol. Biochem. Pharmacol. *104:* 140–215.
3   Fisher, J. W.; Taylor, G.; Porteous, D. D.: Localization of erythropoietin in glomeruli of sheep kidney by fluorescent antibody technique. Nature, Lond. *205:* 611–612 (1965).
4   Busuttil, R. W.; Roh, B. L.; Fisher, J. W.: Localization of erythropoietin in the glomerulus of the hypoxic dog kidney using a fluorescent antibody technique. Acta haemat. *47:* 238–242 (1972).
5   Burlington, H.; Cronkite, E. P.; Reincke, U.; Zanjani, E. D.: Erythropoietin production in cultures of goat renal glomeruli. Proc. natn. Acad. Sci. USA *69:* 3547–3550 (1972).
6   Kurtz, A.; Jelkmann,W.; Sinowatz, F.; Bauer, C.: Renal mesangial cell cultures as a model for study of erythropoietin production. Proc. natn. Acad. Sci. USA *80:* 4008–4011 (1983).
7   Caro, J.; Erslev, A. J.: Biologic and immunologic erythropoietin in extracts from hypoxic whole rat kidneys and in their glomerular and tubular fractions. J. Lab. clin. Med. *103:* 922–931 (1984).
8   Rich, I. N.; Heit, W.; Kubanek, B.: Extrarenal erythropoietin production by macrophages. Blood *60:* 1007–1018 (1982).
9   Jacobs, K.; Shoemaker, C.; Rudersdorf, R.; Neill, S. D.; Kaufman, R. J.; Mufson, A.; Seehra, J.; Jones, S. S.; Hewick, R.; Fritsch, E. F.; Kawakita, M.; Shimaza, T.; Miyake, T.: Isolation and characterization of genomic cDNA clones of human erythropoietin. Nature, Lond. *313:* 806–810 (1985).

10 Lin, F. K.; Suggs, S.; Lin, C. H.; Browne, J. K.; Smalling, R.; Egrie, J. C.; Chen, K. K.; Fox, G. M.; Martin, F.; Stabinsky, Z.; Badrawi, S. M.; Lai, P. H.; Goldwasser, E.: Cloning and expression of the human erythropoietin gene. Proc. natn. Acad. Sci. USA *82:* 7580–7584 (1985).

11 McDonald, J. D.; Lin, F. K.; Goldwasser, E.: Cloning, sequencing, and evolutionary analysis of the mouse erythropoietin gene. Mol. cell. Biol. *6:* 842–848 (1986).

12 Shoemaker, C. B.; Mistock, L. D.: Murine erythropoietin gene: cloning, expression, and human gene homology. Mol. cell. Biol. *6:* 849–858 (1986).

13 Beru, N.; McDonald, J.; Lacombe, C.; Goldwasser, E.: Expression of the erythropoietin gene. Mol. cell. Biol. *6:* 2571–2575 (1986).

14 Bondurant, M. C.; Koury, M. J.: Anemia induces accumulation of erythropoietin mRNA in the kidney and liver. Mol. cell. Biol. *6:* 2731–2733 (1986).

15 Schuster, S. J.; Wilson, J. H.; Erslev, A. J.; Caro, J.: Physiologic regulation and tissue localization of renal erythropoietin messenger RNA. Blood *70:* 316–318 (1987).

16 Scherrer, K.: Isolation and sucrose gradient analysis of RNA; in Habel, Salzmann, Fundamental techniques in virology, pp. 413–432 (Academic Press, New York 1969).

17 Fournier, J.G.; Tardieu, M.; Lebon, P.; Robain, O.; Ponsot, G.; Rozenblatt, S.; Bouteille, M.: Detection of measles virus RNA in lymphocytes from peripheral blood and brain perivascular infiltrates of patients with subacute sclerosing panencephalitis. New Engl. J. Med. *313:* 910–915 (1985).

18 Hume, D. A.; Gordon, S.: Mononuclear phagocyte system of the mouse defined by immunohistochemical localization of antigen F4/80. J. exp. Med. *157:* 1704–1709 (1983).

19 Lacombe, C.; Da Silva, J. L.; Bruneval, P.; Fournier, J. G.; Wendling, F.; Casadevall, N.; Camilleri, J. P.; Bariety, J.; Varet, B.; Tambourin, P.: Peritubular cells are the site of erythropoietin synthesis in the murine hypoxic kidney. J. clin. Invest. (in press, 1987).

20 Bruneval, P.; Da Silva, J. L.; Salzmann, J. L., et al.: Erythropoietin-producing cells in the anemic mouse kidney: in situ hybridization and morphometrical studies (submitted).

21 Tiscer, C. C.; Madsen, K. M.; Anatomy of the kidney; in Brenner, Rector, The kidney, pp. 3–60 (Saunders, Philadelphia 1986).

22 Hawkins, P.; Anderson, S. E.; McKenzie, J. L.; McLoughlin, K.; Beard, M. E.; Hart, D. N.: Localization of MN blood group antigens in kidney. Transplant. Proc. *17:* 1697–1700 (1985).

B. Varet, INSERM U.152, 27, rue du Faubourg St-Jacques,
F-75674 Paris Cédex 14 (France)

Discussion

Caro: I would like to congratulate and your group for the beautiful work you presented. First, what percentage of the interstitium and capillary cells are positive in your hypoxic kidneys, and, second, do you see any preferences around proximal cells or distal tubular cells, and what is the distribution of the positive cells with respect to the type of tubular cells?

Varet: I am not an expert in that field. The percentage of positive cells in the interstitium in the cortex is between 50 and 80% of the cells. We have to do more precise statistical studies on that point. And apparently this number decreases from the cortex to the outer medulla.

Kurtz: Dr. Varet, I would like to ask you a question concerning your technique to count or determine the density of the grains on the cells. You could use this technique to find an answer for the question whether the enhancement or the increase of the message in the hypoxic kidney is due to an enhanced transcription in the erythropoietin-producing cell or to an enhanced recruitment of cells during hypoxia which express the message. Have you done experiments with different hypoxic conditions, for instance, and determined the density of grains on the cells?

Varet: No, we are not trying to do that. We can do it, but it is very hard work and I am not sure that, for the time being, it is the most important question to answer. We are now focusing on the question of the lineage of these cells and after that, perhaps, we will have time to modulate the hypoxic regimen to study that point. It is an important question, but I think that for now the most important point is to make sure that about the lineage of the erythropoietin-producing cells.

Bauer: There are certain points that favor macrophages as possible candidates for EPO production in the kidney. As you probably know, macrophages release very many hemopoetic growth factors, for example, interleukin-1, and they also release some angiogenic factors upon hypoxia. By analogy, the macrophages are certainly not out of the game, I would say.

Varet: The point is that we cannot be sure that these are the only cells which produce erythropoietin. What we can tell you is that in these experiments these cells produce erythropoietin in the hypoxic kidney. Endothelial cells are also, and it is very fascinating, very important and probably more important than macrophages in the production of different growth factors. They produce M-CSF, GM-CSF. The question about macrophages is to determine the specificity of the F4/80 antibody that we used. We believe that previous results are correct and that this antibody is specific for monocytes and macrophages. However, the results we obtained are not exactly the same as those published by Gordon and co-workers in the *Journal of Experimental Medicine* a few years ago. They showed that there are several parts of the murine kidney with numerous monocytic macrophages. We have not found such numerous monocytic macrophages in the murine kidney with this antibody.

Pfäffl: I liked your in situ hybridisation experiments very much and I think there is no question that the kidneys play the key role in the regulation of erythropoietin but on your first slide I have seen at least one organ, the spleen, listed as part of the lymphatic organs. I would like to ask you whether you have done in situ hybridisation in other lymphatic organs like the thymus or the spleen. I missed it on the slides you showed.

Varet: We have not done that, but it was done by Koury and co-workers, I think, and by Beru and Goldwasser. By Northern blot analysis there was no message at all in the spleen of hypoxic animals. From our experience now is clear that it is not useful to use in situ hybridisation if you have negative results by Northern blots. You lose time. To get positive results with the in situ hybridisation, you really have to stress the system. As you have seen in the liver, and I think Caro has the same experience, there is some message by Northern blot analysis, but it was too low to allow an identification of erythropoietin-producing cells by in situ hybridisation.

Kühn: Do you think from a technical point of view that it would be possible in addition to the autoradiography you performed also to use immune peroxidase technique in the same sections to identify endothelial cells by polyclonal antibodies against Wille-brand factor?

Varet: That is exactly what we try to do by double labelling using in situ and immuno-peroxidase or immunofluorescence and there is a technical problem here. You destroy some of the activity you are checking, either by preparing the slide for in situ or either by preparing the slide for immunoperoxidase or any kind of immunolabelling. Then we tried using very potent anti-erythropoietin antibody to see something on these cells by immu-noperoxidase or immunofluorescence, but there is no significant immunolabelling. And it was not really a surprise to us, because using our erythroleukemic cells which produce large amounts of erythropoietin we also got negative results by immunohistochemical tech-niques. It seems that the processing of the protein is very fast in producing cells and apparently the m-RNA stays longer. Then you can get a message for the m-RNA and not for the protein. That is our explanation.

Müller-Wiefel: Did you happen to find any relationship between the intensity of the hepatic erythropoietin production and the age of your mice? And do you have any idea about the adequate stimulants of hepatic eryhtropoietin production, because, from the clinical point of view, there are some reports indicating an increase of hemoglobin during a period of hepatitis, an observation never described during nephritis?

Varet: No, we have not studied that. The only clear-cut point is that hypoxia induces erythropoietin message in the adult liver – that's sure – but if hepatectomy, or any kind of other liver stimulus, is able to do the same thing, we have not tried for the time being. And it is a regulation by hypoxia. There is some clinical evidence that in anephric humans there is still some hypoxic regulation of erythropoietin production. Then the regulation by hypoxia in the liver makes sense and, of course, it will be very interesting to study the liver of humans during hepatitis to look at that. There will probably be an increase after hepatectomy or in regenerating livers, but we have not done the experiment. Our mice were 6 weeks old. We also looked at the fetal liver, but not in an age-dependent fashion, in newborn and adult mice.

Contr. Nephrol., vol. 66, pp. 25–37 (Karger, Basel 1988)

The Role of Erythropoietin in Erythroid Cell Differentiation

Sanford B. Krantz, Stephen T. Sawyer, Ken-Ichi Sawada

Division of Hematology, Department of Medicine, Vanderbilt University School of Medicine and Veterans Administration Medial Center, Nashville, Tenn., USA

Erythropoietin (EPO) is a glycoprotein hormone that is produced in the kidney and acts on bone marrow erythroid progenitor cells to promote development into mature red cells [1]. The principle target cells are the colony-forming units-erythroid (CFU-E), which give rise to single colonies of 8–49 erythroblasts, but EPO also acts on burst-forming units-erythroid (BFU-E), which are more primitive erythroid progenitor cells, to promote development into CFU-E. No effect of EPO on the more primitive, pluri-potential stem cells has been described.

Because EPO is present in picomolar quantities in the serum and urine, it was not purified until 1977, and has only recently become generally available as recombinant human EPO (rhEPO). Initially radioiodination was thought to inactivate the hormone, but since then it has been shown that a ^{125}I-rhEPO ratio of less than 0.6 does not reduce biological activity [2]. Because CFU-E and BFU-E are present at an extremely low frequency of 0.1–1.0%, it has not been possible to study EPO receptors using normal hematopoietic tissues. However, recently the Friend virus that produces 'anemia' (FVA) has been administered to mice to produce a marked splenic accumulation of erythroid cells arrested at a stage of development close to the CFU-E [3]. These cells are easily enriched to provide a population that consists of 95% erythroid progenitor cells, with a yield of 10^8 per infected spleen and a capacity to respond to EPO like CFU-E. In addition, highly enriched human CFU-E have been generated from partially purified blood BFU-E by cell culture with a high concentration of EPO, which has yielded 10^7 erythroid colony-forming cells (ECFC) from 400 ml of blood, with a purity of $70 \pm 18\%$ [4]. These devel-opments have made it possible for us to identify and characterize EPO receptors which is the subject of this report.

Methods

Cell Preparation

FVA cells were generated by administering 10^4 spleen focus-forming units intravenously to CD_2F mice [3]. The spleens were removed 1 week later and contaminant cells were separated by velocity sedimentation at unit gravity. To prepare membranes the cells were suspended in 10 mM KCl/10 mM Tris-HCl, pH 7.4, with 1 mM EGTA and 1 µg/ml leupeptin [5]. The cells were broken with a Dounce homogenizer and the homogenates fractionated by differential centrifugation. The plasma membrane fraction was obtained after equilibrium sedimentation on a discontinuous sucrose gradient.

Human CFU-E were prepared from 400 ml of normal blood collected in heparin [4]. The light density mononuclear cells were gathered from the interface after sedimentation over Ficoll-Hypaque (FH); 1.077 g/cm^3). T cells were then removed by sheep erythrocyte rosette formation and surface immunoglobulin-positive cells were separated by incubation at 4°C for 80 min on plastic dishes coated with affinity-purified sheep anti-human IgG specific for the F(ab)$_2$ fragment. The nonadherent cells were incubated in tissue culture polystyrene flasks overnight at 37°C in a 5% CO_2 atmosphere to remove monocytes by adherence. Nonadherent cells were again removed and were incubated at 70×10^6 cells/ml, at 3°C, with four monoclonal antibodies: 25 µl of CD11b/OKM*1 (20 µg/ml), 25 µl of CD2/OKT*11 (10 µg/ml), 50 µl of CD45R/MY 11 and 50 µl of MY 23 to coat granulocytes, monocytes, colony-forming units-granulocyte-macrophage (CFU-GM), T and B lymphocytes and natural killer cells. After 60 min the cells were washed and incubated at 4°C for 90 min on plastic dishes coated with affinity-purified goat anti-murine IgG. The antibody-negative, nonadherent cells, containing BFU-E, were removed and cultured for 8 days in methylcellulose with complete medium and 2 U/ml rhEPO. The cells were then collected and adherent cells were removed by a 1 h incubation at 37°C in polystyrene flasks. This incubation also removes 90% of the EPO associated with the cells [6]. The nonadherent cells were overlayed on 2 ml of FH [4]. After centrifugation the interface cells were collected and CFU-E were measured by the plasma clot method using rhEPO. ECFC are defined as cells that gave rise to erythroid colonies of 2–49 cells.

Radiolabelled rhEPO

Pure rhEPO, 129,000 U/mg, was iodinated using IODO-GEN [2, 4]. Two micrograms of IODO-GEN in 40 µl of CHCl$_3$ were evaporated onto the wall of a 300-µl conical vial. Two hundred units of the rhEPO and 400 µCi of Na^{125}I were incubated in 50 µl of pH 7 buffer with 10% glycerol and 0.02% Tween 20 for 2 min at 24°C. The mixture was then transferred to a tube containing 0.5 ml PBS, 5 mg KI, 0.02% Tween 20 and 0.1% BSA. The ^{125}I-rhEPO was separated from free ^{125}I by chromatography over a Bio-Gel P6 column equilibrated with PBS containing 0.1% BSA and 0.02% Tween 20. The biological activity of ^{125}I-rhEPO that contained 0.6 molecules of ^{125}I/molecule of rhEPO had greater than 95% retention of biological activity.

Binding of ^{125}I-rhEPO

The cells were incubated with ^{125}I-rhEPO at 37°C in 50–100 µl of binding medium with a cell concentration of not more than 10^7 cells/ml [2, 4]. Binding was terminated by sedimenting the murine cells through 0.5 ml dibutyl phthalate oil, or the human cells

Table I. Binding of ^{125}I-rhEPO to human ECFC

Cells	^{125}I-rhEPO binding, cpm		
	total	nonspecific	specific
FH	79 ± 13	64 ± 12	15 ± 13
ERF[+]	73 ± 20	64 ± 10	9 ± 20
SIg[+]	99 ± 11	109 ± 21	0
AD[+]	101 ± 14	103 ± 8	0
AB[-]	146 ± 24	130 ± 9	16 ± 24
ECFC	189 ± 8	116 ± 4	73 ± 8

[125]I-rhEPO (0.38 nM) was incubated for 20 h at 3 °C with cells obtained by FH density centrifugation, sheep erythrocyte rosette-formation (ERF+), surface immunoglobulin-positive cell enrichment (SIg+), adherence to plastic (AD+), nonadherence after negative panning using a panel of monoclonal antibodies, and generation of ECFC in methylcellulose culture for 8 days. Each value is the mean ± SD of triplicates. The difference between total and nonspecific binding of day 8 ECFC is significant (p < 0,001).

through 0.9 ml of 10% BSA-PBS. The tubes were frozen and the cell pellets were cut off for counting in a gamma counter. Nonspecific binding was determined in the presence of a 20- to 100-fold excess of rhEPO. Specific binding is the difference between total and nonspecific binding. Internalized ^{125}I-rhEPO was measured after removal of external ^{125}I-rhEPO by an acid wash, pH 2.5, prior to cell pelleting. Binding to cell membranes was measured by incubating 10–40 µg of plasma membranes at 37 °C in pH 7.4 buffer with 1 mM EGTA and 0.1% BSA [5]. The binding mixture was applied to 0.2 µm Millipore filters and washed with PBS-BSA. The filters were then counted in a gamma counter.

Cross-Linking of ^{125}I-rhEPO

Cells and membranes bound to ^{125}I-rhEPO were incubated with 0.2 mM disuccinimidyl suberate (DSS) at 0 °C [5]. After 15 min the cross-linking reaction was quenched by addition of ice-cold Tris-HCl, pH 7.4. The cells were centrifuged and resuspended in 0.1% Triton X-100/20 mM Hepes, pH 7.4; the nuclei were pelleted by centrifugation. The supernatant, and ^{125}I-rhEPO cross-labeled to membranes, were boiled for 3 min and analyzed by NaDodSO$_4$/PAGE and autoradiography with Kodak XAR-5 film.

Results

Initial experiments showed specific binding of ^{3}H-EPO and ^{125}I-rhEPO to FVA cells [2, 7] and ^{125}I-rhEPO to human ECFC [4], while no significant specific binding was observed with murine liver, heart, kidney, brain or lung

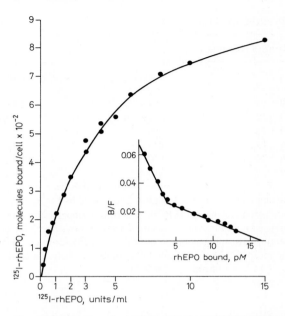

Fig. 1. Scatchard analysis of the binding of ^{125}I-rhEPO to FVA cells. ^{125}I-rhEPO was incubated with FVA cells for 20 h at 4 °C and specific binding was determined as described. Inset: Data replotted by the method of Scatchard. B/F = Bound/free.

[2], or with human T cells, B cells, monocytes or partially purified blood cells that had less than 1% BFU-E (table I). The rate of binding at 37 °C was increased compared to the rate at 3 °C and a stable plateau with twice the amount of binding at 37 °C was present with the human cells, suggesting internalization of the rhEPO at the higher temperature [2, 6]. The binding of ^{125}I-rhEPO was directly proportional to the cell concentration up to 10^7 cells/ml and was reversible for both sets of cells indicating that this was an equilibrium reaction [2, 6, 7]. When the effect of increasing ^{125}I-rhEPO concentrations on specific binding to FVA cells was examined it was evident that saturation of specific binding occurred at 10 U/ml (fig. 1). The Scatchard plot of ^{125}I-rhEPO binding to FVA cells was clearly biphasic suggesting that these cells have two classes of binding sites for rhEPO. Three hundred high affinity receptors with a K_D of 0.09 n*M* were present with an additional 600 receptors that had a K_D of 0.57 n*M*. Plasma membranes prepared from FVA cells had a similar distribution of receptors with almost identical K_D values (fig. 2). A Scatchard plot of ^{125}I-rhEPO binding to human ECFC

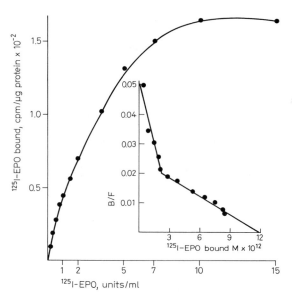

Fig. 2. Effect of concentration of ^{125}I-rhEPO on the binding to plasma membranes from FVA cells. Membranes (2 μg of protein) were incubated for 30 min at 37 °C with ^{125}I-rhEPO and specific binding was determined as described. Inset: Data replotted by the method of Scatchard. B/F = Bound/free. Reproduced from Sawyer et al. [5].

revealed a single class of receptors with 550/ECFC and a K_D of 0.27 n*M* (fig. 3). The correlation coefficient was 0.98.

To determine if endocytosis was present, FVA cells were incubated with ^{125}I-rhEPO at 3 °C and nonbound hormone was then washed away. The cells were then incubated at 37 °C in fresh medium and the distribution of radioactivity amongst the cell surface, interior and medium was determined through the use of an acid wash to remove surface ^{125}I-rhEPO [2]. As shown in figure 4, surface-bound hormone decreased by more than half after 30 min of incubation and at this time approximately 40% of the radioactivity was found inside the cells while 10% was in the medium. Further incubation showed that the internalized EPO declined while medium EPO continued to increase suggesting that the internalized EPO was being expelled from the cells (fig. 4) and analysis of the medium radioactivity indicated that the cell incubation at 37 °C led to the degradation of EPO to iodotyrosine [2]. Internalization of ^{125}I-rhEPO and degradation to iodotyrosine were similarly demonstrated in human ECFC [6].

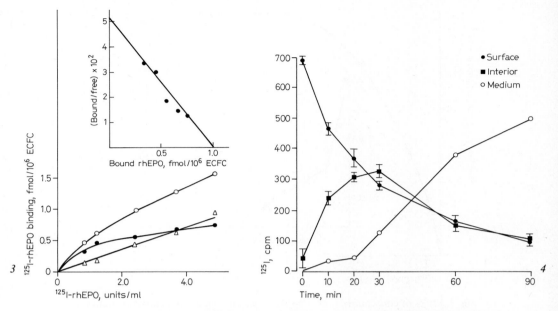

Fig. 3. Effect of ^{125}I-rhEPO concentration on binding to human ECFC. Increasing concentrations of ^{125}I-rhEPO were incubated with 4.0×10^5 day 8 ECFC in 50 μl of medium at 3°C for 8 h. Replicates had a 50-fold excess of unlabeled rhEPO (△) to measure nonspecific binding. Cell-associated ^{125}I-rhEPO was measured (○) and specific binding (●) was calculated. Each point is the mean of duplicates. Replicate cells cultured in plasma clots, in triplicate, gave rise to $75 \pm 11\%$ erythroid colonies. Inset: Scatchard plot by linear regression analysis of the data.

Fig. 4. Time course of endocytosis and degradation of ^{125}I-rhEPO in FVA cells. The cells were incubated with 0.5 unit of ^{125}I-rhEPO/ml for 20 h at 4°C. After unbound hormone was washed away, the cells were warmed to 37°C. At the indicated times, the radioactivity in the medium (○), on the cell surface (●), and in the cell interior (■) were determined as described.

Cross-linking of ^{125}I-rhEPO to FVA cells or plasma membranes demonstrated two major bands that migrated with a molecular mass of a 135 and 120 kilodalton (kDa) in gels with, or without, a reducing agent (fig. 5). These bands, when corrected for the 35 kDa contribution of EPO, were 100 and 85 kDa. Other minor bands were apparent but all disappeared when cross-linking was carried out in the presence of excess EPO [5].

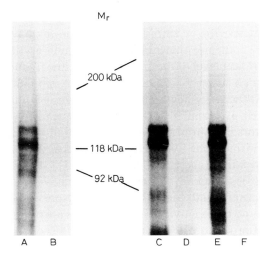

Fig. 5. Cross-linking of ^{125}I-rhEPO to plasma membranes and intact FVA cells. ^{125}I-rhEPO was bound to intact cells (lanes A and B) and plasma membranes (lanes C–F) and cross-linked with 0.2 mM DSS as described. Binding was carried out in the presence of 200 units of unlabeled EPO per milliliter (lanes B, D, and F) and its absence (lanes A, C, and E). The cross-linked material was analyzed by NaDodSO$_4$/PAGE on 5% acrylamide gels in the presence of 2-mercaptoethanol (lanes A–D) and absence (lanes E and F). The positions of molecular size markers (in kilodalton, kDa) are shown. Reproduced from Sawyer et al. [5].

Discussion

The collection of pure murine erythroid progenitor cells following FVA infection has facilitated the study of the mechanisms of action of EPO [8]. It is now known that the hormone enhances $^{45}Ca^{2+}$ uptake into these cells within 1 min [9] and that internalization of the hormone is evident by 10 min, but probably commences much earlier. ^{14}C-2-deoxyglucose uptake into these cells increases within 1 h after the addition of EPO, and total RNA synthesis, measured by ^3H-uridine incorporation increases within 3–4 h [8, 10]. The α- and β-globin gene transcription rate increases by 6 h [10], from a virtually undetectable level, with a concomitant increase in the number of transferrin receptors [11], and this is followed by a prominent wave of hemoglobin synthesis commencing by 12 h. While much has been learned about the time course of these later events that occur as the erythroid progenitor cell mature into late erythroblasts, the second messenger that relays the signal from the EPO receptor to the nucleus and the mechanism of initiation of transcription by specific erythroid genes remain unknown.

The work reported here indicates that murine and human erythroid progenitor cells at the maturation level of the CFU-E have a low frequency of EPO receptors with a high affinity for the hormone. A similar low frequency has been reported for granulocyte-macrophage-colony stimulating factor (GM-CSF) as well as granulocyte-CSF (G-CSF), and may be characteristic of growth factors that promote end-stage maturation [12]. In addition, FVA cells and murine fetal liver cells have a second class of receptors which have a 6- to 8-fold increase in affinity [2, 13]. The higher affinity receptors were not observed in human CFU-E, but very small concentrations of ^{125}I-rhEPO were used to identify these receptors which led to extremely low levels of bound radioactivity. Further studies are necessary with larger cell volumes to compensate for the small ^{125}I-rhEPO concentrations and provide more precise visualization of this area.

The cross-linking experiments demonstrate two bands of 100 and 85 kDa that manifest specific binding to ^{125}I-rhEPO. While our initial studies showed a ratio of 1:2 of the 100-kDa band to the 85-kDa band [5], an increase in proteinase inhibitors has now changed this to a 1:1 ratio, but no combination of up to 13 inhibitors has altered this ratio any further. Cross-linking studies with amounts of ^{125}I-rhEPO that would only bind to receptors of the highest affinity showed an equal increase in radioactivity of both the 85- and 100-kDa proteins indicating that neither is preferentially related to the highest affinity receptors [5]. While one of these bands might not be a receptor protein, but a nearby, innocent bystander protein, our recent work indicates that two bands of similar size are found in human CFU-E and also in the murine placenta. The same observation in different tissues, of different species, reduces the probability that a similar nonreceptor protein would be adjacent to the receptor protein in all of these cases. We, therefore, favor the hypothesis that both bands represent EPO receptor protein(s). Both proteins are found under reduced and nonreduced conditions. While some investigators have reported a large, 200-kDa band under nonreducing conditions, they have not shown a similar degree of labelling for this band and the two bands seen upon reduction [14, 15]. In our experiments the larger band has always had much less radioactivity and has disappeared with sonication and lower concentrations of cross-linker, suggesting that it is an aggregate of ^{125}I-rhEPO and other proteins. The exact relation of the 85- and 100-kDa bands to each other requires further peptide and glycosylation analysis of each and these studies are now underway.

Our studies have also identified internalization and degradation of the ^{125}I-rhEPO as a very early event after its addition to the FVA cells. Chloroquine and NH_4Cl markedly inhibited the degradation suggesting that the site of degradation is lysosomal [2]. While there is no direct evidence of receptor internalization, this generally accompanies the internalization of the hormone and presumably is occurring in CFU-E as well. Since this process only leads to a slight down-regulating of surface EPO receptors [2], despite an extremely fast and extensive endocytosis in which most of the hormone is removed from the cells within 1 h of incubation [2, 6], additional receptors are most likely recycled to the surface after endocytosis, but no data are available concerning this process in erythroid cells.

Since the bone marrow is a large organ with a size equivalent to that of the liver, these studies also indicate that it may make a significant contribution to EPO degradation. Internalization is a dynamic, continuing process and static measurements of the amount of ^{125}I-rhEPO present in the marrow at any time do not adequately represent continuing internalization and degradation. Until equilibrium studies are performed measuring the total turnover of ^{125}I-rhEPO in the marrow, the precise size of the contribution of this organ to EPO degradation will be uncertain. It is also possible that the erythroid progenitor cells modulate EPO levels by a feedback control mechanism whereby EPO levels may be reduced through an increase in erythroid progenitor cells as occurs with macrophages [16]. This is supported by the observation that EPO levels are generally higher in patients with aplastic anemia or red cell aplasia as compared to patients with hyperplastic bone marrows [17], and the reduced half-life of rhEPO that is noted in uremic patients after infusion of the drug for several weeks when erythropoiesis has increased [18].

Internalization of EPO into the CFU-E poses once again the question of how EPO works to trigger the further events of erythroid differentiation. The involvement of several different chromosomes in the initiation of α- and β-gene transcription suggests that a trans-acting factor is regulating specific transcription either as a stimulator or as a de-repressor. This could represent the receptor, the hormone, a fragment of the hormone or the receptor, or another molecular messenger. Whether EPO acts only at the cell surface through the receptor, or inside the cell, with or without the internalized receptor, remains unknown. The key to understanding this process will probably reside in the further characterization and isolation of a pure EPO receptor and further work is now turning in that direction.

Acknowledgements

The authors would like to acknowledge support from Veterans Administration Research Funds and from National Institutes of Health Grants RO1 DK15555, RO1 DK39781 and T32-07186. We also want to thank Ms. Sharon Horn and Ms. Judith Luna for their excellent technical assistance and Ms. Mary Wilson for her assistance in the preparation of the manuscript.

References

1   Spivak, J.: The mechanism of action of erythropoietin. Int. J. Cell Cloning *4:* 139–166 (1986).
2   Sawyer, S.; Krantz, S.; Goldwasser, E.: Binding and receptor-mediated endocytosis of erythropoietin in Friend virus-infected erythroid cells. J. biol. Chem. *262:* 5554–5562 (1987).
3   Koury, M.; Sawyer, S.; Bondurant, M.: Splenic erythroblasts in anemia-inducing Friend disease: A source of cells for studies of erythropoietin-mediated differentiation. J. cell. Physiol. *121:* 526–532 (1984).
4   Sawada, K.; Krantz, S.; Kans, J.; Dessypris, E.; Sawyer, S.; Glick, A.; Civin, C.: Purification of human erythroid colony-forming units and demonstration of specific binding of erythropoietin. J. clin. Invest. *80:* 357–366 (1987).
5   Sawyer, S.; Krantz, S.; Luna, J.: Identification of the receptor for erythropoietin by cross-linking to Friend virus-infected erythroid cells. Proc. natn. Acad. Sci. USA *84:* 3690–3694 (1987).
6   Sawada, K.; Krantz, S.; Sawyer, S.; Civin, D.: Quantitation of specific binding of erythropoietin to human erythroid colony-forming cells. J. cell. Physiol. (submitted, 1988).
7   Krantz, S.; Goldwasser, E.: Specific binding of erythropoietin to spleen cells infected with the anemia strain of Friend virus. Proc. natn. Acad. Sci. USA *81:* 7574–7578 (1984).
8   Krantz, S.; Sawyer, S.; Koury, M.; Bondurant, M.: Use of purified erythropoietin-responsive cells produced by the anemia strain of Friend virus to study the action of erythropoietin; in Rich, Molecular and cellular aspects of erythropoietin and erythropoiesis. NATO ASI Series, vol. H8, pp. 89–102 (Springer, Berlin 1987).
9   Sawyer, S.; Krantz, S.: Erythropoietin stimulates $^{45}Ca^{2+}$ uptake in Friend virus-infected erythroid cells. J. biol. Chem. *259:* 2769–2774 (1984).
10 Bondurant, M.; Lind, R.; Koury, M.; Ferguson, M.: Control of globin gene transcription by erythropoietin in erythroblasts from Friend virus-infected mice. Mol. cell. Biol. *5:* 675–683 (1985).
11 Sawyer, S.; Krantz, S.: Transferrin receptor number, synthesis, and endocytosis during erythropoietin-induced maturation of Friend virus-infected erythroid cells. J. biol. Chem. *261:* 9187–9195 (1986).
12 Metcalf, D.: The molecular biology and functions of the granulocyte-macrophage colony-stimulating factors. Blood *67:* 257–267 (1986).

13   Fukamachi, H.; Saito, T.; Tojo, A.; Kitamura, T.; Urabe, A.; Takaku, F.: Binding of erythropoietin to CFU-E derived from fetal mouse liver cells. Exp. Hematol. *15:* 833–837 (1987).

14   Sasaki, R.; Yanagawa, S.; Hitomi, K.; Chiba, H.: Characterization of erythropoietin receptor of murine erythroid cells. Eur. J. Biochem. *168:* 43–48 (1987).

15   Mayeux, P.; Billat, C.; Jacquot, R.: The erythropoietin receptor of rat erythroid progenitor cells. Characterization and affinity cross-linkage. J. biol. Chem. *262:* 13985–13990 (1987).

16   Bartocci, A.; Mastrogiannis, D.; Migliorati, G.; Stockert, F.; Wolkoff, A.; Stanley, E.: Macrophages specifically regulate the concentration of their own growth factor in the circulation. Proc. natn. Acad. Sci. USA *84:* 6179–6183 (1987).

17   Hammond, D.; Ishikawa, A.; Keighley, G.: The relationship between erythropoietin and severity of anemia in hypoplastic and hemolytic states; in Jacobson, Doyle, Erythropoiesis, p. 351 (Grune & Stratton, New York 1962).

18   Egrie, J. C.; Eschbach, J. W.; McGuire, T.; Adamson, J. W.: Pharmacokinetics of recombinant human erythropoietin (r-HuEpo) administered to hemodialysis (HD) patients (Abstract). Kidney int. *33:* 262 (1988).

Sanford B. Krantz, MD, Professor of Medicine, Chief, Hematology, VA Medical Center, 1310 24th Avenue S., Nashville, TN 37212–2637 (USA)

Discussion

Kurtz: Is iodinated EPO also active in your system?

Krantz: 95% active.

Kurtz: Is the internalization of EPO essential for its biological effect?

Krantz: We cannot dissociate those two events.

Kurtz: What's your feeling?

Krantz: We have no information on that.

Koch: Dr. Krantz, in the beginning of your talk you mentioned a change of half-life after administering EPO to humans for some time. What was the magnitude of this change?

Krantz: It has been reported, perhaps Dr. Eschbach will talk about that. He has an abstract in which the pharmacokinetics show initially a half-life of about 9 h and later after many weeks of EPO treatment a half-life of 6 h.

Varet: Have you tried to add IL-3 instead of EPO on your BFU-E cells to see whether you also get CFU-E?

Krantz: No, we have not done so.

Caro: You find that your saturation was obtained about 1 nm, which is 4 units/ml as you said; however, in your CFU-E cultures the saturation of CFU-E formation is obtained at 0.5 units/ml. Have you any idea why there is a discrepancy between the biological activity and binding activity?

Krantz: At similar low dosage you can see that the biological activity follows binding, but in almost all receptor work there seems to be a large excess of receptors above what the cells actually need and nobody knows why this exists. It is not unique to our system.

Pfäffl: There is evidence that T lymphocytes modulate erythropoiesis. Do you think it is EPO or is it some sort of interleukin-4, -5 or -6?

Krantz: T lymphocytes may play a role in the bone marrow itself. We know for instance that chronic lymphocytic leukemias that consist of T lymphocytes have an effect on modulating erythropoiesis, but I don't think that there has been any correlation with EPO levels.

Pfäffl: What I wanted to hear is whether it is EPO itself or some other modulator which is secreted by the T cells?

Krantz: I cannot think of any study that actually looked at EPO levels in terms of T cell regulation. There have been a lot of direct effects of intact T cells described on the bone marrow itself.

Bauer: Do you have any information on the possible second messenger that might be involved in the EPO action?

Krantz: Well, we have negative results. We have tried to look for increases inositol phosphates, but did not find anything there.

Bauer: Oh good, that's nice at least to know.

Krantz: So, we have no other information.

Bauer: What about cAMP or cGMP?

Krantz: cAMP has no effect on the cells directly, really.

Bauer: And the calcium ionophores? I'am asking this, because with the calcium ionophores one can actually imitate some of their effects of the growth factors in certain cells that are, for example, EGF-dependent.

Krantz: You have to understand that these cells take many hours to develop into the end stage where the markers are studied. Calcium ionophores have no effect on increasing the total development of these cells into hemoglobinized cells. It is possible they might have a very early action if we had an early marker to observe.

Kurtz: What is the effect of phorbol esters on the differentiation of these cells?

Krantz: On these cells they have no effect.

Kurtz: This means stimulation of the protein C kinases has no effect with all its consequences.

Krantz: We have no evidence that it has any effect. We tried phorbol esters on these cells. Phorbol esters have been shown to have effects on some murine cell culture lines, but those lines are not responsive to EPO.

Winearls (London): Your purification procedure is laborious. I wondered whether you managed to stain in the final product with the antibody to the leukocyte common antigen, whether this would simplify the purification by just eliminating them at an early stage?

Krantz: We haven't tried that. It is not so laborious but simply an application of sequential methods. It all takes place in one day.

Bauer: What kind of specific activity of the EPO do you assume for the Scatchard analysis, I mean, how active is the EPO once it is iodinated?

Krantz: In the early days of iodinating EPO when Dr. Goldwasser was doing this he was heavily iodinating it in order to use it for the radioimmunoassay. When he tested the biological activity it was not active. It turns out that if you iodinate it to a much lesser extent, so that you have less than one molecule of iodine per molecule of EPO, you then see good biological activity. So we try to keep it less than one molecule. There are four iodotyrosines on EPO. If you iodinate at a frequency so that not more than one is bound, then you have good biological activity. At this level of iodination two thirds of the erythropoietin molecules are radioactive.

Bauer: And you also told us that you are getting EPO receptors in the placenta that are similar to the receptors we were seeing on the CFU cells. As far as I know, the EPO does not cross the placental barrier.

Krantz: Well, I think the biological studies many years ago seemed to suggest that it did not cross, but Drs. Koury, Bondurant and Sawyer at our place have injected radioactive EPO into the maternal mice and you can find it on the other side of the placenta in the fetus.

Bauer: As the original molecule?

Krantz: As the original molecule by size.

Contr. Nephrol., vol. 66, pp. 38–53 (Karger, Basel 1988)

Molecular Biology of Erythropoietin

P. Hirth[a], *L. Wieczorek*[b], *P. Scigalla*[b,1]

[a]Abteilung Genetik und [b]Produktentwicklung Therapeutika,
Boehringer Mannheim GmbH, Mannheim, FRG

Human erythropoietin (EPO) was first isolated and purified to homogeneity from urine of patients with aplastic anemia [1]. Using such material in the polycythemic mouse model, the bioactivity, i. e. the stimulation of differentiation of red blood cells, was demonstrated [2–4]. After the EPO gene had been cloned and expressed, material became available for both biochemical analysis and clinical trials. A number of recent biochemical studies describe the structure-function relationship of the EPO molecule.

Cloning of EPO Genes

The cloning of human EPO sequences has been described [5–7]. To briefly review the strategy employed: human urinary EPO was purified to homogeneity and tryptic fragments were isolated and subjected to N-terminal amino acid analysis. After retrotranslation, two different pools of mixed oligonucleotide probes were used to screen a human genomic library. A fragment containing EPO-coding sequences was isolated and then used to screen a cDNA library that was constructed from poly-A+ RNA isolated from human fetal liver. Figure 1 shows the complete cDNA sequence of human EPO. The amino acid sequence deduced from the nucleic acid sequence was in good agreement with the data obtained from sequencing the urinary EPO [5]. The protein is synthesized as pro-form that contains a 27 amino acid leader which is processed during secretion. The N-terminus of the mature protein is alanine as confirmed by amino acid sequencing.

[1] We thank our cooperative partners Genetics Institute, Cambridge, Mass., for their support in the preparation of this manuscript.

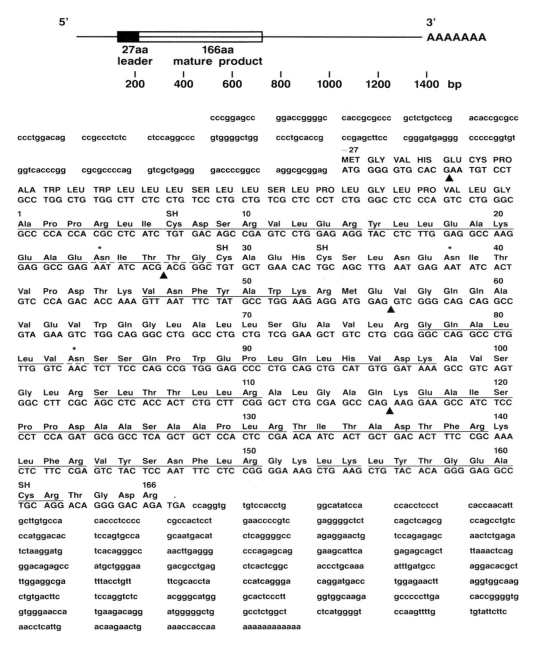

Fig. 1. Complete cDNA sequence of human EPO. From [5].

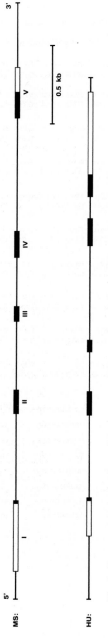

Fig. 2. Structural organization of the mouse (MS) and human (HU) EPO gene. From [7].

```
tctagactcagcctagttgtttctgatctaaatccctgctcaagacaaggatgCTCCCACCCCC CACACACCCCC gcccccaggtgttccggcgcccaactttcata GGTCAATTA tccttacgtcagcctaggcttaccttcc    150
cg CAAATCT ctcagatggcaccccctggtct ACCCTCTCTGGAAATCAGAACCTCCCCCCCCCAAAACCCCTGACGGCG TGTGTGCCTGGAACAGCCTGCTCACCCCAGCAAGCACCAGA CCCAGGCGTCCTGCCCCTTGCTCTG    300
ACCCCAGGTGGCCCCCACCTCTGGGCAGCCCTCAGCGACACACAGCTTCACCCCACCCCACCCGACCACGCACACATGGTGGCACACATGCTGATAAACATCCCGACCCCCGGACCGGAGCCAACCCTCGCCGGTGGCTGTGTCT    450
CACTGTGTTCCCGAACGGACCCCCTTGGCCAGGGCACCGGTCCCCACCTCTGCCCGCGCCCGTCTGGACAGTGACCACCTTCTTCCCAGGCTAGTGGGGTGATCTGGCCCTACAGAACTTCCAAGGATGAAGACTTGCAGCGTGGACACTGGCC    600
CAGCCCCGGGTCGCCTAAGGAGCTCCGGCAGCTCCGGCGCGGAG ATG GGG GTG CCC G gtgagtactcacaggctaaggaccctgtgacctcaggctcctgtttgagtaaggattacatctaaagctattggtcaggaaaccgac    744
                                            ATG GGG GTG CAC G
cgtgttcaaggacctgcgactctccaaggatcaaggaagaggagggggtggggcagcctccacgtgcactaaggggtttggggagccccctgtgaatgcactagggatccagaacagggacaaaattaggatttgggggag    894
atgaggcggctgctgtgtgagtgaaagctgctaaaggaattacctgcgtcaggagtccctgcttccaggatctgcgcgcaccccagtgaagtttggccgagaagtggatgccggtcgtgctgggggtggggtgtgca    1044
gcgcgggaggggattgaatgaaggccactcaggcagacagccaagtgcaaggtcggggtcagcagagactaaaggcagagggggtcgctgagccaagcagagggggtggggcgccgccccctctcggcctcacctcagc    1194
ctgcctttcttcag AA  CGT  CCC  ACC  CTG  CTT   TTA  CTC  TCC   TTG  CTA  CTG  ATT   CCT   CTC  GGC CTC  TGT   GCT  CCC  CCA  CGC   CTC   ATC  TGC  GAC  AGT  CGA  GTT  CTG    1310
              AA  TGT  CCT  GCC* CTG  TGG   CTT  CTC  CTG  TCC   CTG  CTG  CTC   CCT  CTG  GGC  CTC  CCA  GTC  CTG  GGC   GCC  CCA  GTC  CTC  ATC  TGT  GAC  AGC  CGA  GTC  CTG
              AA  TGT  CCT  GCC* CTG  TGG   CTT  CTC  CTG  TCT   CTG  CTC  TCG   CTG  CTC  GGC  CTC  CCA  GTC  CTC  GGC   GCC  CCA  CGC  CTC  ATC  TGT  GAC  AGC  CGA  GTC  CTG
GAG AGG TAC  ATC  TTA  GAG  GCC  AAG  GAG  GCA  GAA  AAT   GTC  ACG gtaagctccctggcccaccaaagaaagaaactggttcagggatctgggaattggggttccttccggaactaccttagggacaagataag    1446
GAG AGG TAC  CTC  TTG  GAG  GCC  AAG  GAG  GCC  GAG  AAT   ATC  ACG
GAG AGG TAC  CTC  TTG  GAG  GCC  AAG  GAG  GCC  GAG  AAT   GTC  ACG
atgtttaaccccttaaacctctttcatccccccgacaagaatgataaaactgggcagggggattggccagttggtaaagagttgcaagacgccctaggttcgattccaagtactgcacaaacatttggttggcataaac    1596
ctacaatcccagtgttggaggtggtgaggaagtgaggagaattcaagtgatcctagctacatatccaagtgtgaggccaacctgggttacctgaaactatgtctaaaataaaagaatagacaaagctggtggttcccaaagcatgccg    1746
```

```
gtaaaattcaaagacagagtgtctgatggctttttgtggacatttgacctggggctgtgtcttttag ATG GGT TGT GCA GAA GGT CCC AGA CTG AGT GAA AAT ATT ACA GTC CCA GAT ACC AAA GTC 1874
                                                                    ACG GGC TGT GCT GAA CAC TGC AGC TTG AAT GAG AAT ATC ACT GTC CCA GAC ACC AAA GTT
                                                                    ATG GGC TGT TCC GAA AGC TGC AGC TTG AAT GAG AAT ATC ACC GTC CCA GAC ACC AAA GTT

AAC TTC TAT GCT TGG AAA AGA ATG GAG gtgagttgcattgtgtctggtccctgtccttgtccccatctgtctgtctgtctgaccgcccatccatgcccccaccctctccacccttggttcttagaggttggtgggtctcat 2015
AAT TTC TAT GCC TGG AAG AGG ATG GAG
AAC TTC TAT GCC TGG AAG AGG ATG GAG

tttcacatctttatagtgtgggagaaaatatcagagacaatggttcatgggatagagtagctcataatatattcattcattcattcattcattcattcattcagtaaaccttactgcttgcttttctgttccttctttcagtcctgtata 2165

atagccagggaggatagggaatgacattggttggctgtttctaagtctttgactcccctag GTG GAA GAA CAG GCC ATA GAA GTT TGG CAA GGC CTG TCC CTG CTC TCA GAA GCC ATC CTG CAG GCC 2292
                                                              GTC GGG CAG CAG GCC GTA GAA GTC TGG CAG GGC CTG GCC CTG CTG TCG GAA GCT GTC CTG CGG GGC
                                                              GTC GGG CAG CAG GCT GTA GAA GTC TGG CAG GGC CTG GCC CTG CTC TCA GAA GCT GTC CTG CGG GGC

CAG GCC CTG CTA GCC AAT TCC TCC CAG CCA CCA GAG ACC CTT CAG CTT CAT ATA GAC AAA GCC ATC AGT GGT CTA CGT AGC CTC ACT TCA CTG CTT CGG GTA CTG GGA GCT 2403
CAG GCC CTG TTG GTC AAC TCT TCC CAG CCG TGG GAG CCC CTG CAG CTG CAT GTG GAT AAA GCC GTC AGT GGC CTT CGC AGC CTC ACC ACT CTG CTT CGG GCT CTG GGA GCC
CAG GCC GTG TTG GCC AAC TCT TCC CAG CCT TTC GAG CCC CTG CAG CTG CAC ATG GAT AAA GCC ATC AGT GGC CTT CGC AGC ATC ACC ACT CTG CTT CGG GCG CTG GGA GCC

CAG gtgagtgtgagtgcctgtggaccctgctacttgcccttctacaggatgcactaagaactgttgaaagaaccctgaggtctgagccagggagagctcagcggggaaatgagctcgatgctaagcctgatgccctgggacccacaagc 2552
CAG
CAG

tgaaagtcctctaagcgaattaatgtaataacaaatttaaaacaaagactactgacagctcagtctgcggagatgaatcaagggatggcatgctggctgcacaagtgtgaggagccaagttcgatctccagcacttccatttaaaaaaaa 2702

agaaaatgagatgaggtggaaggtacacatgatcccagagctggggaggcagactcgcaaggactcctgggactcactggccagccagtctggatcagtgagctccaggctttactaagagagatgctgtctcgaaacattagacgcagg 2852

gctggaggcatggctcaatgattaggagcgcttgctgctcttgcagggttcaatacc cagcatccatatcgggtgcctcatagctgcctttacaccc atctctagggaatctaagggtgtattctggatgccccgggcacctgcatacat 3002

tcacatccacatatccaaataaaaataatgtggagactgcctgaagaagacacacctctgcacacaccgacctcccattctggaccaggtcacatcttatctgtgagccctccacactccagtgacatcctattctctcttgacag AAG 3151
                                                                                                                                                        AAG
                                                                                                                                                        ---

GAA TTG ATG TCG CCT CCA GAT ACC ACC CCA CCT GCT CCA CTC CGA ACA CTC ACA GTG GAT ACT TTC TGC AAG CTC TTC CGG GTC TAC GCC AAC TTC CTC CGG GGG AAA CTG 3262
GAA GCC ATC TCC CCT CCA GAT GCG GCC TCA GCT GCT CCA CTC CGA ACA ATC ACT GCT GAC ACT TTC CGC AAA CTC TTC CGA GTC TAC TCC AAT TTC CTC CGG GGA AAG CTG
GAA GCC ATC TCC CTC CCA GAT GCG GCC TCG GCT GCT CCA CTC CGA ACC ATC ACT GCT GAC ACT TTC TGC AAA CTC TTC CGA GTC TAC TCC AAT TTC CTC CGG GGA AAG CTG

AAG CTG TAC ACG GGA GAG GTC TGC AGG AGA GGG GAC ACG TGACATGCTGCTGCCACCGTGGTGGACCGACGAACTTGCTCCCCGTCACTGTGTCATGCCAACCCTCCACCACTCCCAACCCTCATCAAACGGGTCAT 3399
AAG CTG TAC ACA GGG GAG GCC TGC AGG ACA GGG GAC AGA
AAG CTG TAC ACG GGG GAG GCC TGC AGG AGA GGG GAC AGA

TACCTTCTTACCAGTCTGTCCCATGGACACTCCAGCACCAGCAGTGACATCCTCGGGGCCAGAAGAACTTCCCAGAGCTCCATTCTGAAATCTAAAGATGTCGCTGGACAAGCCCGAGGCCCAGAGAAGAAGAGCCTCAGAATCAGCTCG 3549

gatttgtttaggtttttttttttttttgaaacaggaaggtctcacatagcccaggctggcctggaactcgctgtgtagttaaaggacagcattgaattcctgatctttccgcttctggttctcaagtgctgagattacaggcaccctg 3699

tccccgtttatggggtgttagagatggaagctggggcttcctgcatgctaggcaagcactctattaactgaactatgtcctcagctcccagagaccggacttagacctcagggacagagatgtccaaactcaactagtgccctgccagaa 3849

ctgtaaccagtcccctctccccacccccacaggacaagctt 3891
```

Fig. 3. Nucleotide sequence of the mouse EPO gene and coding sequences of monkey and human EPO. Coding regions are indicated by triplet spacing, and the corresponding sequences from human monkey genes are given on the first and second lines below each mouse line, respectively. Intervening sequences are printed in small letters. From [7].

Translation termination occurs after arginine at position 166. Canonical sequences for N-glycosylation are at positions asparagine 24, 38 and 83. There is one site in the molecule for O-glycoxylation at position serine 126. The molecular weight of the protein portion of the molecule was calculated to be 18,490 daltons.

The structural organization of the mouse and human EPO gene is shown in figure 2. EPO information is contained within five exons. In humans, a relatively long 5′ untranslated region and part of the leader peptide is located in exon I, whereas the genetic information of the mature EPO is within exons II, III and V. Figure 2 also shows that the structural organization is very similar for the two genes; spacing of exons, however, is clearly different.

The DNA sequence of the mouse EPO gene is given in figure 3 with the coding sequences grouped into triplets. Below the mouse sequence the coding sequences of human and monkey EPO are aligned.

A comparison of the three genes on the amino acid sequence level is shown in figure 4 [7]. Human and monkey EPO share 92% homology, human and mouse have 80% amino acids in common whereas monkey and mouse have 82% homology. The number and the relative positions for N-linked carbohydrates are conserved in all three species whereas the serine at position 126 is only present in human and monkey EPO. O-glycosylation thus does not seem to interfere with bioactivity and receptor binding, at least in the mouse, as O-glycosylated human EPO is fully active [7, 8].

Structure predictions based on the amino acid sequence can be made by computer according to Chow and Fasman [9]. A comparison of the hypothetical structures is shown in figure 5. In all molecules the cysteines in positions 7 and 161 are used to form a disulfide bridge, thus connecting the very N- with the very C-termini. The two other cysteines (positions 29 and 33) in monkey and in human EPO can be used to form a bridge and a small loop. Although in mouse the cysteine at position 33 is missing a similar structure could be established with the help of the replacing proline in that position.

Fig. 4. Amino acid sequence of mammalian EPOs. The sequence of the mouse (MS) protein is presented along with differences from this sequence in the human (HU) and monkey (MO) proteins of the first and second lines below the mouse sequence, respectively. Numbering is from the amino terminus of the human protein. The asterisks (*) indicate the sites of potential N-linked glycosylation. From [7].

Fig. 5. Comparison of putative structures of mouse, monkey and human EPO. From [7].

```
        -27                                    +1                              * 25
MS:  NH₂-M-G-V-P-E-R-P-T-x-L-L-L-L-L-S-L-L-L-I-P-L-G-L-P-V-L-C-A-P-P-R-L-I-C-D-S-R-V-L-E-R-Y-I-L-E-A-K-E-A-E-N-V-
HU:        H  C  AW W         S L            G                               L               I
MO:        H  C  AW W         VSL            PG                              L

                                             50                              75
MS:  T-M-G-C-A-E-G-P-R-L-S-E-N-I-T-V-P-D-T-K-V-N-F-Y-A-W-K-R-M-E-V-E-E-Q-A-I-E-V-W-Q-G-L-S-L-L-S-E-A-I-L-
HU:      T        H C S  N                                G Q   V         A         V
MO:      S        S C S  N                                G Q   V         A         V

                                             100                             125
MS:  Q-A-Q-A-L-L-A-N-S-S-Q-P-P-E-T-L-Q-L-H-I-D-K-A-I-S-G-L-R-S-L-T-S-L-L-R-V-L-G-A-Q-K-E-L-M-S-P-P-D-T-T-
HU:  R G       V           W P  V     V            T         A I         A A
MO:  R G   V               F P      M             I T        A     x A I    L    A A

                                             150                    166
MS:  P-P-A-P-L-R-T-L-T-V-D-T-F-C-K-L-F-R-V-Y-A-N-F-L-R-G-K-L-K-L-Y-T-G-E-V-C-R-R-G-D-R-COOH
HU:  S A     I    A     R          S                          A    T
MO:  S A     I    A                S                          A
```

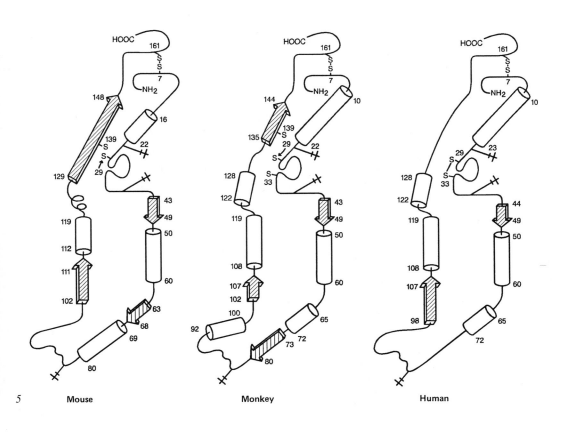

Mouse   Monkey   Human

According to figure 5, the differences in amino acid sequence do not seem to cause a dramatic change in the overall structure of these molecules. Relatively stronger conservation of structure seems to be in the organization of the 60 first amino acids when α-helix, β-sheets, glycosylation sites and S-S bridging are compared.

Expression of Human EPO

Since subsequent studies show that in order to be effective in vivo the recombinant EPO should be closely related to its natural counterpart, a mammalian expression system is the only practical approach. The human EPO cDNA was ligated after some modifications into an expression vector and placed under the control of a heterologous promotor that allows continuous synthesis. This vector also contains a selectable marker (dhfr). As a host cell system, Chinese hamster ovary cells were used that are deficient in dihydrofolate reductase. This cell line has been shown to be a suitable host for heterologous expression of human proteins as not only high producer cell lines can be established but probably even more important secondary modifications of proteins such as glycosylation are very similar to those in humans [10].

The expression vector described was transfected into these cells and EPO-producing colonies were isolated. Subsequently the EPO-coding sequences were coamplified with methotrexate to yield high producer cell lines. For actual EPO production the CHO cells can be grown in large fermenters where the EPO is secreted into the culture fluid out of which it can be purified.

Description of Recombinant EPO with Emphasis on Aspects That Are Important for Its Clinical Use

When EPO of this source was used in bioassays such as the in vitro mouse spleen assay [11] or in the polycythemic mouse model [12], EPO activity could be demonstrated.

To analyze the protein moiety of recombinant EPO, a quantitative amino acid composition analysis was performed, the result of which is given in table I. The actual numbers of moles of each amino acid are presented as average of several produced lots of recombinant human EPO (rhEPO). Also

Table I. Amino acid composition of recombinant and urinary human EPO [from 15]

	Recombinant human EPO, average of 5 lots mol	Urinary human EPO, WHO reference standard mol
Asn + Asp	11.9	11.8
Thr	10.5	9.8
Ser	9.2	7.7
Glu + Glu	19.0	19.0
Pro	8.0	8.5
Gly	9.0	9.9
Ala	18.9	19.3
Cys	3.4	–
Val	10.4	11.0
Met	0.6	0.5
Ile	4.6	5.0
Leu	23.3	24.5
Tyr	3.9	3.9
Phe	4.0	3.7
His	2.0	2.1
Lys	7.9	8.4
Trp	n.d.	n.d.
Arg	12.0	12.2

n.d. = Not determined.

in table I, the numbers of moles of amino acid of urinary EPO, that is used as WHO reference standard, are shown for comparison. The data obtained are in very good agreement and demonstrate that the correct material is synthesized. Based on the cDNA prediction, however, arginine is underrepresented by 1 mol in both recombinant and urinary EPO. One possible explanation for these results is that the COOH-terminal arginine predicted at position 166 is missing from the purified product. However, DNA sequence analysis of the EPO-coding segment of the production cell line indicated that no mutation had occurred. Therefore, COOH-terminal processing of modification could be an explanation. To test this hypothesis, a COOH-terminal EPO fragment produced after digestion with endoproteinase Lys-C was subjected to N-terminal analysis (table II). The data in table II show that COOH-terminal arginine can be detected in neither the recombinant EPO nor in the urinary EPO. These data have meanwhile been confirmed by FABMS analysis [13]. As all other amino acids of the terminal

Table II. N-terminal sequence analysis of carboxy-terminal endoproteinase Lys-C peptide of recombinant and urinary human EPO (international standard) [from 15]

Recombinant human EPO			Urinary human EPO		
cycle	amino acid	pmol	cycle	amino acid	pmol
1	Leu	120	1	Leu	85
2	Tyr	170	2	Tyr	84
3	Thr	68	3	Thr	43
4	Gly	130	4	Gly	45
5	Glu	105	5	Glu	42
6	Ala	120	6	Glu	43
7	Cys	n.d.	7	Cys	n.d.
8	Arg	46	8	Arg	27
9	Thr	45	9	Thr	16
10	Gly	64	10	Gly	17
11	Asp	10	11	Asp	8
12	(Asp)	8	12	(Asp)	6
13	(Asp)	6	13	(Asp)	4
14	–		14	–	–
15	–		15	–	–

n.d. = Not determined.

fragment were observed as predicted in the expected ratios, the COOH-terminal processing and removal of arginine seem to be very specific.

Digestion of recombinant and urinary EPO with endoproteinase Lys-C and fractionation of the resulting fragments on HPLC allows a complex analysis not only of the protein moiety but also of other modifications. Figure 6 shows that similar patterns were obtained for both types of molecules indicating that on the basis of this experiment they cannot be distinguished.

Another important aspect of EPO is its carbohydrate moiety which amounts to about half the molecular weight. The carbohydrates are absolutely essential for the bioactivity of EPO in vivo. Intensive analyses were carried out to determine the carbohydrate composition of rhEPO. Table III shows the types of sugars found and their molar concentrations per mol protein. The presence of N-Ac Gal is an indication for an O-glycosylation. Figure 7 shows the structures of recombinant EPO from CHO cells as

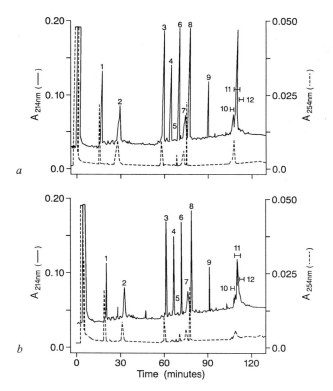

Fig. 6. Separation of fragments produced by endo-Lys C of rhEPO *(a)* and urinary human EPO *(b)*. From [13].

Table III. Carbohydrate composition of recombinant EPO[1]

Sugar	Lot, mol sugar/mol protein				
	P5	P6	P7	P8	P9
Fucose	3.1 ± 0.5	3.0 ± 0.3	2.7 ± 0.2	2.9 ± 0.7	3.0 ± 0.2
Mannose	10.2 ± 0.3	10.9 ± 0.4	9.6 ± 0.4	10.7 ± 0.8	11.0 ± 0.5
Galactose	13.3 ± 0.8	12.9 ± 0.6	12.1 ± 0.9	12.9 ± 0.8	13.2 ± 0.7
NAcGal	0.7 ± 0.1	0.7 ± 0.1	0.7 ± 0.1	1.0 ± 0.1	0.7 ± 0.1
NAcGlc	16.2 ± 1.1	15.0 ± 0.3	16.4 ± 0.3	16.8 ± 0.2	15.8 ± 0.5
Sialic acid	14.8 ± 0.1	14.2 ± 0.8	14.6 ± 0.4	14.6 ± 0.1	14.7 ± 0.5

[1] Data based on an analysis of 21 samples; values expressed represent the mean ± SD. From Genetics Institute, Cambridge, Mass. [unpublished].

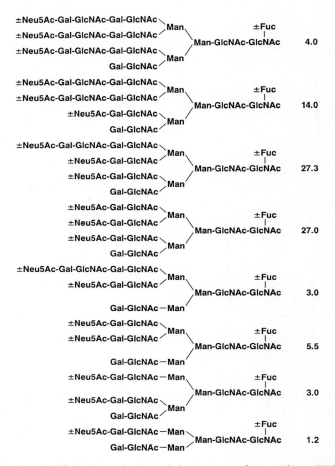

Fig. 7. N-linked carbohydrate chain structure of recombinant EPO. From [14].

published by Sasaki et al. [14] in 1987. There are very few glycosylation sites occupied with bi-antennaries, about 10% are occupied with tri-antennaries and the majority are tetra-antennaries containing an average of 3 mol of sialic acid each.

The effect of sialic acid content on the bioactivity of EPO is shown in figures 8 and 9. In figure 8, EPO was treated with different concentrations of sialidase and then assayed in the mouse spleen assay (in vitro system). Clearly the removal of terminal sialic acid residues enhanced the specific

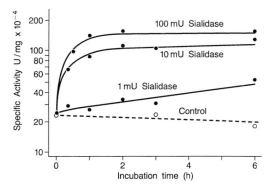

Fig. 8. Change in biological activity of EPO after desialylation in vitro. From N. Ochi and T. Kawaguchi [unpublished].

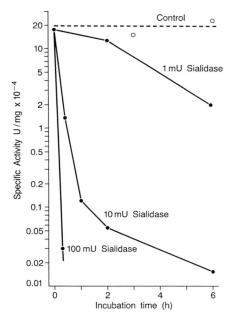

Fig. 9. Effect of desialylation on the biological activity of EPO in vivo. From N. Ochi and T. Kawaguchi [unpublished].

activity by up to a factor of 8. However, when the corresponding EPO samples are assayed in vivo (polycythemic mouse) a dramatic decrease in specific activity is observed (fig. 9). This is due to the fact that desialylated EPO is cleared very efficiently by the asial receptor in the liver. The data further indicate that sufficient sialic acid residues are present in recombinant EPO to give a significant response. Whether recombinant and urinary EPO can be compared in this respect remains unclear as urinary EPO has experienced exposure to serum for an unknown amount of time and it has been secreted by the kidneys where metabolic processes could potentially occur.

References

1   Miyake, T.; Kung, C. K.-H.; Goldwasser, E.: Purification of human erythropoietin. J. biol. Chem. *252:* 5558–5564.
2   Goldwasser, E.: Erythropoietin and the differentiation of red blood cells. Fed. Proc. *43:* 2285–2292 (1975).
3   Wang, F. F.; Kung, C. K.-H.; Goldwasser, E.: Some chemical properties of human erythropoietin. Endocrinology *116:* 2286–2292 (1985).
4   Lai, P. H.; Everett, R.; Wang, F. F.; Arakawa, T.; Goldwasser, E.: Structural characterization of human erythropoietin. J. biol. Chem. *261:* 3116–3121 (1986).
5   Jacobs, K.; Shoemaker, C.; Rudersdorf, R.; Neill, E. F.; Kaufman, R. J.; Mufson, A.; Seehra, J.; Jones, S. S.; Hewick, R.; Fritsch, E. F.; Kawakita, M.; Shimaza, T.; Miyake, T.: Isolation and characterization of genomic and cDNA. Nature, Lond. *313:* 806–810 (1985).
6   Lin, F. K.; Suggs, S.; Lin, C.-H.; Browne, J.; Smalling, R.; Egrie, J.; Chen, K.; Fox, G.; Martin, F.; Stabinsky, Z.; Brdrawi, S.; Lai, P.-H.; Goldwasser, E.: Cloning and expression of the human erythropoietin. Proc. natn. Acad. Sci. USA *82:* 7580–7584 (1985).
7   McDonald, J. D.; Lin, F. K.; Goldwasser, E.: Cloning, sequencing and evolutionary analysis of the mouse erythropoietin. Mol. cell. Biol. *3:* 842–848 (1986).
8   Shoemaker, C. B.; Mistock, L. D.: Murine erythropoietin gene: cloning, expression and human gene homology. Mol. cell. Biol. *6:* 849–858 (1986).
9   Chou, P. Y.; Fasman, G. D.: Empirical predictions of protein conformation. A. Rev. Biochem. *47:* 251–267 (1987).
10 Kaufman, R. J.; Wasley, L. C.; Spiliotes, A. J.; Grossels, S. D.; Latt, S. A.; Larsen, G. R.; Kay, R. M.: Coamplification and coexpression of human tissue-type plasminogen activator and murine dihydrofolate reductase sequences in Chinese hamster ovary cells. Mol. cell. Biol. *5:* 1750–1759 (1985).
11 Krystal, G.: A simple microassay for erythropoietin based on ³H-thymidine incorporation into spleen cells from phenylhydrazine treated mice. Exp. Hematol. *11:* 649–660 (1983).

12   Erslev, A. J.: in Williams, Beutler, Erslev, Lichtmann, Hematology, 3rd ed., pp. 1634–
      1635 (McGraw-Hill, New York 1983).
13   Recny, M. A.; Scoble, H. A.; Kim, Y.: Structural characterization of natural human
      urinary and recombinant-DNA-derived erythropoietin. Identification of des-Arg 166
      EPO (submitted).
14   Sasaki, H.; Bothner, B.; Dell, A.; Fukuda, M.: Carbohydrate structure of erythro-
      poietin expressed in Chinese hamster ovary cells by a human erythropoietin cDNA. J.
      biol. Chem. *262:* 12059–12076 (1987).

Dr. Peter Hirth, Boehringer Mannheim GmbH, Abteilung Genetik,
Nonnenwald 2, D-8122 Penzberg (FRG)

Discussion

Winearls (London): I understand that if you do isoelectric focussing on erythropoietin, there is more than one species. I wonder whether you could comment?

Hirth: May I see the third-last slide? Look at the structure of this molecule and
compare this structure here. This is a biantennary. This molecule has one residue of
sialic acid and, as you all know, sialic acid is heavily negatively charged. If you look at
this molecule, for example, you have at least three molecules of sialic acid residues
linked to the asparagine, which gives an enormous difference in charge and this change
would cause a very different behavior in isoelectric focussing gels, because the isoelectric
point is clearly shifted towards an acidic pH. And this explains why you might get a
heterogeneous population of molecules in isoelectric focussing gels. Does this answer
your question?

Winearls: Yes, can you tell us whether isoelectric focussing of native, urinary erythropoietin is the same as recombinant?

Hirth: I am not in the position to comment on that.

Kurtz: Is there any information about which part of the molecule interacts with the
receptor?

Hirth: Well, you can only speculate in terms of what is conserved in the molecule and
we know that the mouse or the human molecule works in the mouse and that this structure is
very much conserved. We only can speculate so far, but we have to wait until further data
emerge from the cross-linking studies that are probably already underway and look at what
kind of contacts are made between the two molecules. Well, we do know that some
antibodies raised against the N-terminals do not neutralise. That means that part of the
molecule is probably not involved in receptor binding.

Varet: CHO cells are malignant cells. Is there no problem to use a product from
malignant cells to therapy in humans?

Hirth: If you purified the product and made sure that all the substances you would
consider hazardous are removed, I think it is pretty safe.

Varet: A second question: There is no CAT box and no TATA box on that gene.
Can you comment about the hypothesis about the promotion on the regulation of the
gene?

Hirth: A lot of promoters, regulatory regions, or 5-flanking region of genes transcribed by polymerase II actually do contain a TATA box. Some people also call that the promoter. But there are also a number of genes that do not contain these sequences but are still regulated in a very complex fashion. The LDL receptors are a very good example. HMG CoA-reductase also does not contain a TATA box. As far as I know, in terms of regulatory elements they have been screened for metal-responsive elements, for glucocorticoid-responsive elements which are known to exist, but no correlation was found.

Müller-Wiefel: Is there any evidence to suppose a difference between urine and serum erythropoietin concerning their molecular structure?

Hirth: We do not have data and so it is pure speculation. I should mention that the concentrations of erythropoietin in the blood are somewhere in the pg/ml range and so far nobody has managed to isolate it to a decent homogeneity in sufficient quantities to allow analysis. We do not know. All we do know is that when you compare the protein composition, termini of the protein and the sugar composition they are very similar, although there are small differences.

Bauer: Perhaps I may add a comment to Dr Varet's question. Scientists in Glasgow at the Betson Institute cloned a number of genes that are expressed coordinately during erythroid maturation and they conclude from their analyses that the TATA box is absent in the so-called housekeeping genes, and the TATA box is present in the what they call luxury genes. The globin gene, for example, would be a luxury gene. EPO, therefore, is not considered to be a luxury gene, with regard to the TATA box. But I think you are of the opinion that the presence or absence of the TATA box does not say anything?

Hirth: No, we know that the erythropoietin gene is expressed and, as I mentioned, there are other genes that do not contain a TATA box.

Bauer: There is also no polyadenylation site present.

Hirth: The polyadenylation site has not been identified yet. What we do know is that erythropoietin m-RNA contains a poly-A tail. That was demonstrated during cDNA synthesis. It is just that we do not know the sequence.

Stummvoll (Linz): Until now I believed EPO had 166 amino acids. You now show that it has only 165. Is this correct? What is the difference between the urinary and plasmatic EPO? Is there a difference in glycosylation and molecular weight between urinary and plasmatic EPO.

Hirth: To answer your first question: The 166 amino acids were historical and based on the cDNA prediction. It was only when erythropoietin was carefully analysed and characterized that it was found that one amino acid was missing, and this initiated studies looking at the urinary EPO and the result was that also in the urinary EPO this C-terminal amino acid was missing. Now to your second question concerning the carbohydrate composition. I am not sure I really understand what you mean. I tried to show data that glycosylation is very similar in both types of molecules.

Stummvoll: The molecular weight of erythropoietin in plasma is 40,000, whereas you mentioned 18,000 for the recombinant EPO and the urinary EPO.

Hirth: 18,000 is only based on the amino acid content and I mentioned that half of the molecule is carbohydrate. How do you determine the molecular weight of such a structure? You obviously cannot use SDS gels because you only get apparent molecular weights.

Stummvoll: So you do not think there are differences between the plasma and the urinary EPO.

Bauer: Not to my knowledge.

Hirth: I do not know. As long as we cannot isolate it, it remains speculation.

Bauer: The urinary EPO is, of course, purified according to its activity in the polymouse. So, anyhow, you are selecting for molecules that are biologically active. Now I have one question with regard to the specific activity of the various EPO preparations because there are numbers around between 70,000 and 250,000 per mg which makes a difference by a factor of more than three.

Hirth: I am asked not to discuss the specific activities of these molecules and I am sorry I cannot give you an answer.

Bauer: Maybe, Dr. Krantz has some information on that?

Krantz: I am sorry, I do not.

Contr. Nephrol., vol. 66, pp. 54–62 (Karger, Basel 1988)

Erythropoietin Assays and Their Use in the Study of Anemias

Jaime Caro, Allan J. Erslev

Cardeza Foundation for Hematologic Research, Department of Medicine, Thomas Jefferson University, Philadelphia, Pa., USA

Erythropoietin (EPO) is a glycoprotein hormone which regulates the rate of proliferation and differentiation of erythroid precursors in the bone marrow [1]. It is part of a complex feedback system (fig. 1) which ultimately adjusts the size of the red cell mass to the demand of oxygen by the tissues. It is primarily synthesized in the kidney in response to anemic or hypoxic hypoxia and although extrarenal sites also exist, they probably do not represent more than 10% of total EPO production. Although the mechanism of oxygen sensing has not been clearly established, it is known that exposure to acute hypoxia determines the rapid accumulation in the kidney of specific EPO mRNA which precedes the synthesis and secretion of the active hormone [2].

EPO was first purified to homogeneity by Miyake et al. [3] and shown to have an apparent molecular weight of about 38,000 daltons and a specific activity of about 74,000 units/mg. The recent cloning of the human [4] and mouse [5, 6] EPO gene has indicated that the EPO molecule contains 166 amino acids with a peptide molecular weight of 18,000 daltons. There are three N-glycosylation sites and with the carbohydrate content the total molecular weight is believed to be around 34,000 daltons.

EPO Measurements

The concentration of EPO in plasma can be measured by three general techniques: in vivo bioassay, in vitro bioassay and radioimmunoassay. The in vivo bioassay measures the biologic activity of EPO in the intact animal and it is considered the reference assay against which the other assays are compared. EPO measurements are usually expressed in units or milliunits of the reference Standard B prepared under the auspices of and distributed by

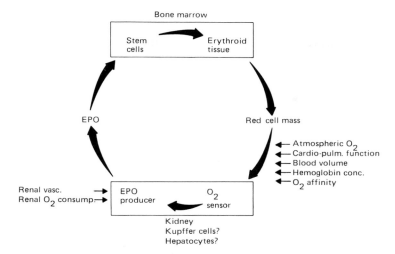

Fig. 1. Schematic representation of the feedback system that regulates red cell production.

the World Health Organization. The Standard B was prepared from urine of anemic patients and has a specific activity of about 5 units/mg [7]. A unit was originally defined as the erythropoietic activity elicited in rats after the injection of 5 μM of $CoCl_2 \cdot 6H_2O$.

The in vivo bioassay utilizes polycythemic mice by either hypertransfusion or preexposure to hypoxia for a period of 2 weeks [8]. These polycythemic animals have a very low endogenous level of EPO and can be utilized for the measurement of exogenously injected EPO. The effect of EPO on red cell production is measured by the incorporation of ^{59}Fe into circulating erythrocytes (see fig. 2). The lowest limit of sensitivity with this assay is about 50 mU and will not detect the erythropoietic activity found in normal plasma. Fortunately, EPO is quite heat-resistant, and by acid heat extraction it is possible to prepare a low protein extract which can then be concentrated 40–60 times. Utilizing this concentration technique, Erslev et al. [9] were able to determine the concentration of EPO in normal human plasma and found it to be about 8 mU/ml with a range between 3 and 18 mU/ml of plasma. Unfortunately, this concentration technique requires large amounts of plasma which are not readily available from most patients except from those with polycythemia.

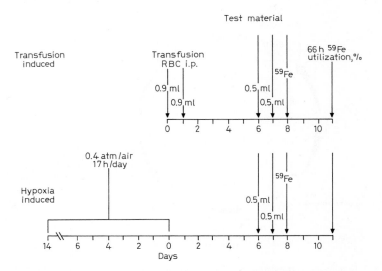

Fig. 2. Schematic representation of in vivo bioassay of EPO.

Numerous in vitro bioassays have been designed and shown to be of use in measuring EPO titers [10]. These assays are based on short-term cultures of erythroid tissue derived from marrow, spleen or fetal livers. The erythropoietic effect is measured by the incorporation of ^{59}Fe into newly formed heme, the uptake of ^{3}H-thymidine as a measure of cellular proliferation or the stimulation of CFU-E formation in semisolid media. The main problem with in vitro techniques is the presence of some poorly defined inhibitors in human sera and the nonspecific stimulatory effect of other growth factors in these in vitro systems.

The successful purification of human EPO by Miyake et al. [3] and the subsequent cloning of the EPO gene has allowed the development of sensitive and specific radioimmunoassays [11, 12]. These assays utilize radio-labelled pure EPO and antibodies developed against either pure or impure EPO, EPO oligopeptides or fusion proteins. Radioimmunoassays have the potential of measuring nonbiologically active asialo-EPO. However, there have been no confirmed reports on significant discordance between bioassays and radioimmunoassays. Figure 3 shows a typical radioimmunoassay displacement curve showing the parallel between Standard B and EPO obtained from normal or anemic patients. The lower limit of sensitivity of radioimmunoassay is about 2–4 mU/ml of sample.

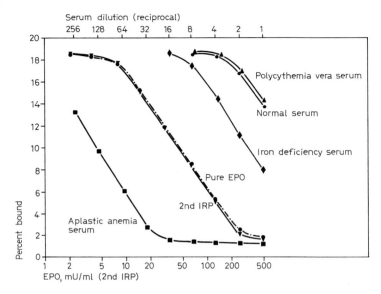

Fig. 3. Radioimmunoassay of human EPO. Standard curve with International Standard B (2nd IRP) and serial dilutions of normal and anemic human sera [from 11].

EPO in Anemias

Simple Anemias. As expected from the feedback circuit depicted in figure 1, a decrease in the concentration of hemoglobin will produce a marked increase in circulating levels of EPO. Figure 4 shows the inverse correlation between hematocrit and EPO levels in patients with simple anemias not complicated by renal disease or inflammatory processes. EPO titers increase exponentially in relation to the degree of the anemia and values up to 1,000 times normal values are observed in severe anemias [13].

Hemolytic Anemias and Anemias Secondary to Chronic Inflammation. Figure 5a and b depicts the EPO levels observed in patients with sickle cell disease and in patients with anemia secondary to rheumatoid arthritis [13]. As can be seen in the figure, the levels of EPO are well within the expected levels seen in simple anemias suggesting that in these conditions the mechanisms controlling EPO production are functioning normally.

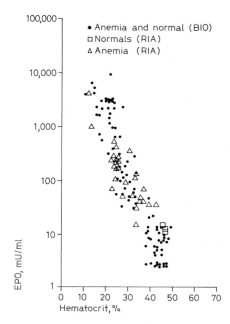

Fig. 4. Relationship between hematocrit and EPO levels measured both by bioassay and radioimmunoassay in patients with anemias not complicated by renal or chronic diseases [from 13].

Anemia of Chronic Renal Disease. In contrast with the above conditions, EPO levels in anemic uremic patients are inappropriately low for their degree of anemia as shown in figure 6 [14]. Anephric patients have the lowest level which fit with the clinical observation of the severity of the anemia in these patients. This inappropriate response to hypoxia in chronic renal patients appears to be important in the pathogenesis of the anemia of renal disease since administration of exogenous EPO can correct the anemia in these patients [15].The abnormal relationship between hematocrit and EPO titers is normalized after successful renal transplantation as recently shown by Besarab et al. [16].

Conclusion

The study of EPO titers in patients with anemias has confirmed the regulatory role of EPO in the control of red cell production. Simple anemias

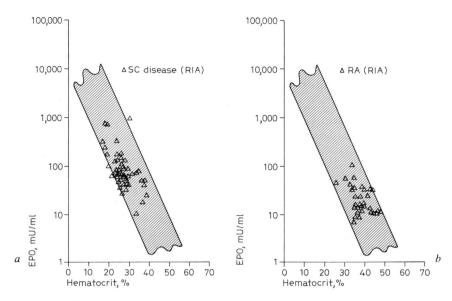

Fig. 5. EPO levels measured by radioimmunoassay in patients with sickle cell anemia *(a)* or anemia secondary to rheumatoid arthritis *(b)* [from 13].

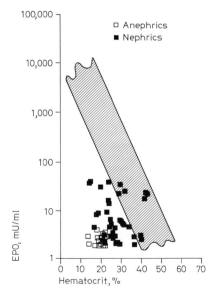

Fig. 6. EPO titers in patients with anemia secondary to chronic renal diseases.

have shown a characteristic inverse relationship between hematocrit and plasma EPO levels. This relationship is maintained in hemolytic anemias or anemias of chronic inflammatory process. In contrast, patients with anemia of chronic renal disease show inadequate production of EPO, suggesting a preponderant role of EPO deficiency in the genesis of this anemia. Replacement therapy seems then the appropriate therapy for the anemia of renal failure. In all other anemias, EPO may be of benefit by stimulating further red cell production, but its use should be considered more as a pharmacologic treatment than a physiologic replacement.

References

1   Spivack, J.: The mechanism of actions of erythropoietin. Int. J. Cell Cloning *4:* 139–166 (1986).
2   Schuster, S.; Wilson, J.; Erslev, A. J.; Caro, J.: Physiologic regulation and tissue localization of renal erythropoietin messenger RNA. Blood *70:* 316–318 (1987).
3   Miyake, T.; Kung, C.; Goldwasser, E.: Purification of human erythropoietin. J. biol. Chem. *252:* 5558–5564 (1977).
4   Jacobs, K.; Shoemaker, C.; Rudersdorf, R.; Neill, S.; Kaufman, R.; Murson, A.; Leehra, J.: Jones, S.; Hewick, R.; Fritsh, E.; Kawakita, M.; Shimizu, T.; Miyake, T.: Isolation and characterization of genomic and cDNA clones of human EPO. Nature, Lond. *313:* 806–810 (1985).
5   Shoemaker, C.; Mitsock, L.: Murine EPO gene: cloning, expression and human gene homology. Mol. cell. Biol. *6:* 849–858 (1986).
6   McDonald, J.: Lin, F.; Goldwaser, E.: Cloning, sequencing, and evolutionary analysis of the mouse erythropoietin gene. Mol. cell. Biol. *6:* 842–848 (1986).
7   Annable, L.; Cotes, P. M.; Mussett, M. V.: The second international reference preparation of erythropoietin, human, urinary, for bioassay. Bull. Org. mond. Santé *47:* 99–112 (1972).
8   Kazal, L. A.; Erslev, A. J.: The measurement of erythropoietin. Ann. clin. Lab. Sci. *5:* 91–97 (1975).
9   Erslev, A. J.; Caro, J.; Kansu, E.; Miller, O.; Cobbs, E.: Plasma erythropoietin in polycythemia. Am. J. Med. *66:* 243–247 (1979).
10 Dunn, C. D. R.; Lange, R. D.: Erythropoietin: assay and characterization; in Roaths, Topical reviews in hematology, pp. 1–32 (Wright, Bristol 1980).
11 Birgegard, G.; Miller, O.; Caro, J.; Erslev, A. J.: Serum erythropoietin levels by radioimmunoassay in polycythaemia. Scand. J. Haematol. *29:* 161–167 (1982).
12 Garcia, J.; Sherwood, J.; Goldwasser, E.: Radioimmunoassay of erythropoietin. Blood Cells *5:* 405–419 (1979).
13 Erslev, A. J.; Wilson, J.; Caro, J.: Erythropoietin titers in anemic, nonuremic patients. J. Lab. clin. Med. *109:* 429–433 (1987).
14 Caro, J.; Brown, S.; Miller, O.; Murray, T.; Erslev, A. J.: Erythropoietin levels in uremic nephric and anephric patients. J. Lab. clin. Med. *93:* 449–458 (1979).

15   Eschbach, J. W.; Egrie, J. C.; Downing, M. R.; Browne, J. K.; Adamson, J. W.:
      Correction of the anemia of end-stage renal disease with recombinant human eryth-
      ropoietin. New Engl. J. Med. *316:* 73–78 (1987).
16   Besarab, A.; Caro, J.; Jarrell, B. E.; Francos, G.; Erslev, A. J.: Dynamics of erythro-
      poiesis following renal transplantation. Kidney int. *32:* 526–536 (1987).

Jaime Caro, MD, Cardeza Foundation for Hematologic Research,
Thomas Jefferson University, 1015 Walnut Street, Philadelphia, PA 19107 (USA)

Discussion

Kühn: I would like to ask you what your opinion is about the mechanism that causes patients with sepsis or infection to have usually lower EPO levels in relation to their anemia than other patients?

Caro: Well, as I've mentioned, that is a complicated issue. We have done experiments in rats where starvation decreased the level of EPO significantly. We have also done that in humans. If you have a normal volunteer fasting for 4 days (as we have done), the EPO level goes down from normal to below normal values. I think that is probably contributing to a significant level. There may be other variations, you know, in shock, or in patients with sepsis, there are cardiovascular adaptations. We do not know what kind of effects they would have on kidney blood flow distribution, on oxygen utilization in the kidney, etc. We do not know what is happening there. So I do not know the explanation, but it is certainly true that these very sick patients do have lower EPO levels than expected.

Bommer: Perhaps I missed it. What was the immunosuppressive therapy in your transplant patients? Was it ciclosporin or azothioprine?

Caro: We have used both ATG and ciclosporin. We had a recent paper, I think in *Kidney International* last month, where the data is broken down according to each treatment. I think this is using both combined.

Schurek (Hannover): In rheumatoid arthritis, did you look for differences between treated and untreated patients, treated with prostaglandin synthesis inhibitors or not?

Caro: I think we only looked for corticoid steroids. I do not know whether prosta-glandin inhibitors make a difference. We did not find any difference whether patients were treated with steroids or not.

Koch: What happens to the EPO levels in those uremic patients who have slightly elevated levels when you transfuse them? Are they going down?

Caro: At the time we did those studies we did not have radioimmunoassays available. It was too much to do plasmaphoresis in those patients before and after transfusion. So we don't have that data.

Koch: So you never investigated this?

Caro: Whether these were completely autonomous or not? I would think that a percentage of that EPO production is likely to be autonomous, based on the posttransplant studies.

Winearls (London): Those studies have actually been done in dialysis patients. When they are bled or when they have the EPO levels measured after bleeding and after transfusion, there seems to be quite a good feedback mechanism, but it's all rather truncated. It was in *Kidney International* this year.

Böning: Did you ever investigate the effects of normal physiological variations like bedrest or physical activity on EPO?

Caro: No, we haven't.

Grützmacher: May I answer this. We examined this and unter circadian rhythm, exercise, orthostatic stress and supine bedrest saw no real change, only differences of less than 10%.

Koch: What assay?

Grützmacher: It is our Frankfurt bioassay using the fetal mouse liver assay which we think is very sensitive.

Bauer: It may be sensitive, but exactly what you measure is really unknown. Do you agree?

Grützmacher: I would disagree. There are exact rules using bioassays and I can assure you that you can apply these rules on a bioassay as represented by the fetal mouse liver cell assay. There is absolute parallelity between the standard dilution curve and the samples measured.

Caro: I have reservations about in vitro assays but I think you are using internal controls for a patient before and after exercise, and using the same serum, it is probably valid to do it. I think the most difficult thing is when one tries to extrapolate from work with the in vitro cultures, like, you know, trying to see whether tumors or cell lines are producing EPO. There are some growth factors that simulate EPO activity in vitro and not being EPO and there is some nonspecific toxicity in human serum that can also affect the assay.

Bauer: You have to take care of very many things in such an assay. Let me ask you about the sensitivity of your polycythemic mouse assay. You were saying that the hypertransfused mouse is more sensitive than the exhypoxic mouse?

Caro: What I say is that the base level of a hypertransfused mouse is much more stable. It is always below 0.2% iron incorporation and in the exhypoxic polycythemic mouse the base level is usually a little bit higher and you have more variation. So when you are talking of measuring low levels of EPO, I think the polycythemic mouse hypertransfused is a better assay.

Bauer: But this depends on how much you cut down the endogenous production of EPO. What happens if you use, for example, hypobaric in comparison to isobaric hypoxia? With isobaric hypoxia we in Zürich are getting down to zero percent iron incorporation as base level.

Caro: If you can consistently bring down your iron incorporation I think it is probably okay, but most of the assays have a 1–3% baseline. And when you are talking about a 3% baseline and you measure a 0.5% increase in incorporation, I mean, you cannot do very sensitive assays.

Varet: The question could be relevant for nephrologists using recombinant EPO. Have you compared the EPO level in patients with the same degree of anemia and without erythroblasts in their bone marrow compared to patients with erythroblasts in their bone marrow?

Caro: No, we haven't. It is a very interesting thing. Some people postulate that the half-life of EPO, as Dr. Krantz mentioned, may be related to destruction by erythroblasts in their bone marrow. It used to be said that aplastic anemia patients would have higher levels than other patients. But in our hands we do not see this difference very clearly.

Contr. Nephrol., vol. 66, pp. 63–70 (Karger, Basel 1988)

Modern Aspects of the Pathophysiology of Renal Anemia

Joseph W. Eschbach, John W. Adamson

University of Washington, Seattle, Wash., USA

The association of anemia with renal failure has been recognized for over 100 years since Richard Bright first described the manifestations of chronic renal failure. Little was understood about this anemia until 30 years ago when erythropoietin (EPO), the hormone that regulates erythropoiesis, was demonstrated to be of renal origin [1]. However, it has been only in the past several years, since molecular biology has provided recombinant human EPO (rhEPO) [2, 4], that we are now on the threshold of not only better understanding the pathophysiology of the anemia, but also of correcting it [5–7].

The significance of anemia in renal failure is probably greater than previously appreciated. Approximately 200,000 people are receiving chronic dialysis therapy in the world, and over 75% of these patients are moderately to severely anemic with hematocrits of less than 30. Anemia is probably the major reason why only a minority of patients with end-stage renal disease are rehabilitated with chronic dialysis. Up to 50% require periodic red cell transfusions to prevent symptoms of severe hypoxia [8]. However, transfusion therapy is incomplete, transient and fraught with the risk of infection, development of cytotoxic antibodies and further erythroid suppression [9]. By correcting anemia relatively rapidly with rhEPO and observing the various symptom-complex improvements, it is apparent that anemia results in more disabling symptoms than previously appreciated [10].

Mechanisms of the Anemia

The major mechanisms that contribute to anemia include shortened red cell survival, decreased EPO production, blood loss because of the qualitative platelet defect present in uremia, and possibly retained inhibitors or toxic metabolites that inhibit erythropoiesis. Other mechanisms may develop in the dialysis patient and aggravate anemia. These include iron and folate deficiency, aluminum toxicity, osteitis fibrosa associated with severe hyperparathyroidism, transfusion-induced erythroid suppression, and any cause of hemolysis, such as hypersplenism.

EPO deficiency appears to be the major cause of the anemia. Although it has been known for many years that any cause of hypoxia is a stimulus to the kidney to produce EPO, only recently have studies indicated the tubular or capillary origin of EPO secretion in the kidney [11, 12]. Under normal circumstances, a low level of circulating EPO (10–30 mU/ml plasma) is capable of maintaining a stable red cell mass [13]. However, plasma EPO levels, as measured by radioimmunoassay, may increase 100- to 200-fold in response to impaired oxygen delivery to the normal kidney [13]. Therefore, in the presence of moderate to severe renal disease, the kidney has a blunted response to anemia or other forms of impaired oxygen delivery, and is unable to increase EPO production (as reflected by an inability to increase plasma EPO levels). Hence, the severity of anemia is often directly correlated with the extent of renal insufficiency.

Inhibitors of erythropoiesis have been postulated to be a major cause of anemia for many years and, if present, might blunt the effect of EPO therapy. Several different cell systems are inhibited by an uremic environment: lymphocyte response or proliferation to mitogens, and in vitro erythropoiesis. In general, when murine marrow cells are cultured in the presence of growth factors including EPO, the addition of uremic human serum reduces the number of erythroid progenitor cells (colony-forming units-erythroid; CFU-E). Three substances have been incriminated as possible inhibiting solutes: parathyroid hormone, spermine and ribonuclease. There are also in vivo observations that suggest that toxic metabolites may inhibit erythropoiesis. When the serum of anemic dialysis patients was concentrated, bioassay for EPO indicated that about 40% of the patients had EPO levels higher than those found in normal, nonanemic humans. These observations suggested that inhibitors of erythropoiesis might have prevented normalization of the patients' hematocrits [14]. There have been several attempts to infuse human EPO into anemic patients with chronic renal failure. The first reported attempt utilized human urine that was toxic and failed to result in any reticulocytosis [15]. The infusion of EPO-rich plasma from a patient with aplastic anemia into several patients with renal failure did not result in erythroid stimulation as measured by reticulocytosis, unless the degree of uremia was mild [16]. Anemia has also corrected itself with the induction of continuous ambulatory peritoneal dialysis [17], suggesting to many that the more porous peritoneal membrane allows for better removal of erythroid inhibitors, if present. However, anemia also spontaneously improves in many hemodialysis patients, but less than 5% achieve a normal hematocrit.

Hemolysis, although mild, occurs to a variable degree in renal failure. Red cell survival, normally 120 days, as measured by several different radioisotopic techniques, is between one half to two thirds of normal by the time advanced renal failure develops. The mechanism for the hemolysis is thought to be due to some retained solute(s) because red cell survival is corrected if uremic red cells are transfused into a nonuremic milieu. Most reports fail to document any normalization of red cell survival with dialysis.

Newer Insights

In vitro Studies. In an attempt to confirm whether parathyroid hormone (PTH) was inhibitory of erythropoiesis, we studied the effect of purified PTH on CFU-E growth in the presence of EPO [18, 19]. No inhibition was seen. Spermine is not elevated in dialysis patients [20], and although inhibitory of CFU-E, spermine also inhibits granulocyte progenitor cells (CFU-GM), suggesting that its inhibitory effect is not specific [21]. Ribonuclease-induced CFU-E inhibition occurs only when unphysiologic amounts of ribonuclease are added to the culture media [22]. If mouse, rat or dog erythroid marrow cells are used in culture, the uremic inhibition of CFU-E is nonspecific; that is, there is also inhibition of in vitro granulopoiesis and megakaryocytopoiesis [23], yet leukocyte and platelet numbers in the blood of patients with renal failure are usually normal. Of even greater significance though is that when an entirely autologous in vitro culture system was employed, no inhibition of erythroid progenitor cells was observed with uremic sera in the presence of EPO [24].

Animal Models. In an attempt to circumvent the possible unphysiologic nature of the in vitro studies, various animal models of chronic renal failure with anemia have been established. The animals were then infused with animal or human EPO. In general, most models have shown variable responses to heterologous EPO. We developed an entirely homologous model, using the sheep, which was surgically manipulated to create a stable degree of renal failure and anemia. When these animals were infused with EPO-rich sheep plasma, this not only corrected the anemia, but their response to the EPO was identical in both the normal and uremic states, indicating that there was no inhibition to the action of EPO [25]. In vitro evaluation of the effect of normal or uremic sheep serum on normal or uremic marrow cells also failed to detect any inhibition of the EPO effect on CFU-E growth [26].

Recombinant Human Erythropoietin. It is difficult to know whether animal models are analogous to the human situation and so the only way to conclusively decide whether uremic inhibitors of erythropoiesis exist is to study humans. Fortunately, the human gene for EPO has now been success-fully cloned and expressed by cultured Chinese hamster ovary cells [2–4]. The recombinant hormone, isolated from the culture medium, has been shown to have the same amino acid sequence and biologic and immunologic properties as the natural urinary hormone [27]. rhEPO is active when infused into anemic dialysis patients at doses of 50 units/kg or more, three times a week [5]. The fact that almost all treated patients respond in a predictable manner [28], and a dose-response type curve is observed [5], adds further evidence that uremic inhibitors are unlikely to be present, but if they are, they can easily be overcome by rhEPO. Studies now underway in the anemic patient with advancing renal failure indicate that rhEPO is just as effective in the nondialyzed state as in the hemodialysis patient, implying that dialysis does not remove any erythropoietic inhibitor. However, until rhEPO is infused into normal subjects and responses (reticulocytosis and ferrokinetics) to equal amounts of rhEPO are compared to those in the uremic patients, we cannot say conclusively whether or not erythropoietic inhibitors exist in vivo. However, that information should be forthcoming in the near future.

Conclusion

The pathophysiology of the anemia of chronic renal failure, although multifactorial, now appears to be mainly due to the deficiency in adequate production of the renal hormone, EPO, by the diseased kidney. While mild hemolysis persists it does not prevent normalization of the hematocrit with rhEPO therapy, and if inhibitors exist, their physiologic significance is minimal.

References

1 Jacobson, L.; Goldwasser, E.; Fried, W.; Plzak, L.: Role of the kidney in erythropoiesis. Nature, Lond. *179:* 633–634 (1957).

2 Jacobs, K.; Shoemaker, C.; Rudersdorf, R.; Neill, S. D.; Kaufman, R. J.; Mufson, A.; Seehra, J.; Jones, S. S.; Hewick, R.; Fritsch, E. F.; Kawakita, M.; Shimizu, T.; Miyake, T.: Isolation and characterization of genomic and cDNA clones of human erythropoietin. Nature, Lond. *313:* 806–810 (1985).

3 Lin, F. K.; Suggs, S.; Lin, C. H.; Browne, J. K.; Smalling, R.; Egrie, J. C.; Chen, K. K.; Fox, G. M.; Martin, F.; Stabinsky, Z.; Badrawi, S. M.; Lai, P. H.; Goldwasser, E.: Cloning and expression of the human erythropoietin gene. Proc. natn. Acad. Sci. USA *82:* 7580 (1985).

4 Egrie, J. C.; Browne, J. K.; Lai, P.; Lin, F.-K.: Characterization and biological effects of recombinant human erythropoietin. Immunobiology *172:* 213–224 (1986).

5 Eschbach, J. W.; Egrie, J. C.; Downing, M. R.; Browne, J. K.; Adamson, J. W.: Correction of the anemia of end-stage renal disease with recombinant human erythropoietin. Results of a combined phase I and II clinical trial. New Engl. J. Med. *316:* 73–78 (1987).

6 Winearls, C. G.; Oliver, D. O.; Pippard, M. J.; Reid, C.; Downing, M. R.; Cotes, P. M.: Effect of human erythropoietin derived from recombinant DNA on the anemia of patients maintained by chronic haemodialysis. Lancet *ii:* 1175–1178 (1986).

7 Bommer, J.; Alexiou, C.; Muller-Buhl, U.; Eifert, J.; Ritz, E.: Recombinant human erythropoietin therapy in haemodialysis patients – dose determination and clinical experience. Nephrol. Dial. Transplant *2:* 238–242 (1987).

8 Crowley, J. P.; Nealey, T. A.; Metzger, J.; Pono, L.; Chazan, J. A.: Transfusion and long-term hemodialysis. Archs intern. Med. *147:* 1925–1928 (1987).

9 Eschbach, J. W.; Adamson, J. W.; Cook, J. D.: Disorders of red blood cell production in uremia. Archs intern. Med. *126:* 812–815 (1970).

10 Eschbach, J. W.; Adamson, J. W.: Recombinant human erythropoietin: Implications for nephrology. Am. J. Kidney Dis. (in press).

11 Caro, J.; Erslev, A. J.: Biologic and immunologic erythropoietin in extracts from hypoxic whole rat kidneys and in their tubular glomerular fractions. J. Lab. clin. Med. *103:* 922–931 (1984).

12 Besareb, A.; Caro, J.; Erslev, A.: Erythropoietin synthesis in the isolated perfused kidney. Proc. Xth Int. Congr. Nephrol., 1987.

13 Garcia, J. F.; Ebbhe, S. N.; Hollander, L.; Cutting, H. O.; Miller, M. E.; Cronkite, E. P.: Radioimmunoassay of erythropoietin: Circulating levels in normal and polycythemic human beings. J. Lab. clin. Med. *99:* 624–635 (1982).

14 Caro, J.; Brown, S.; Miller, O.; Murray, T.; Erslev, A. J.: Erythropoietin levels in uremic nephric and anephric patients. J. Lab. clin. Med. *93:* 449–457 (1979).

15 Van Dyke, D.; Keighley, G.; Lawrence, J.: Decreased responsiveness to erythropoietin in a patient with anemia secondary to chronic uremia. Blood *22:* 838 (1963).

16 Essers, U.; Muller, W.; Heintz, R.: Effect of erythropoietin in normal man and in patients with renal insufficiency. Proc. Eur. Dial. Transplant Ass. *11:* 398–402 (1974).

17 Zappacosta, A. R.; Caro, J.; Erslev, A.: Normalization of hematocrit in patients with

end-stage renal disease on continuous ambulatory peritoneal dialysis. Am. J. Med. *72:* 53–57 (1982).

18 Delwiche, F.; Garrity, M. J.; Powell, J. S.; Robertson, R. P.; Adamson, J. W.: High levels of the circulating form of parathyroid hormone do not inhibit in vitro erythropoiesis. J. Lab. clin. Med. *102:* 613–620 (1983).

19 McGonigle, R. J. S.; Wallin, J. D.; Husserl, F.: Deftos, J. L.; Rice, J. C.; O'Neill, W. H.; Fisher, J. W.: Potential role of parathyroid hormone as an inhibitor of erythropoiesis in the animal of renal failure. J. Lab. clin. Med. *104:* 1016–1026 (1984).

20 Spragg, B. P.; Bentley, D. P.; Coles, G. A.: Anaemia of chronic renal failure. Polyamines are not raised in uraemic serum. Nephron *38:* 65–66 (1984).

21 Caro, J.; Hickey J.; Erslev, A. J.: Is spermine the uremic erythropoietic inhibitor? Clin. Res. *31:* 309A (1983).

22 Freedman, M. H.; Saunders, E. F.; Cattran, D. C.; Rbin, E. Z.: Ribonuclease inhibition of erythropoiesis in anemia of uremia. Am. J. Kidney Dis. *2:* 530–533 (1983).

23 Delwiche, F.; Segal, G.; Eschbach, J.; Adamson, J.: Hematopoietic inhibitors in chronic renal failure. Lack of in vitro specificity. Kidney int. *23:* 641–648 (1986).

24 Segal, G. M.; Eschbach, J. W.; Egrie, J. C.; Stueve, T.; Adamson, J. W.: The anemia of end-stage renal disease: Progenitor cell response. Kidney int. (in press).

25 Eschbach, J.; Mladenovic, J.; Garcia, J. F.; Wahl, P. W.; Adamson, J. W.: The anemia of chronic renal failure in sheep. Response to erythropoietin-rich plasma in vivo. J. clin. Invest. *74:* 434–441 (1984).

26 Mladenovic, J.; Eschbach, J. W.; Garcia, J. F.; Adamson, J. W.: The anaemia of chronic renal failure in sheep: Studies in vitro. Br. J. Haemat. *58:* 491–500 (1984).

27 Egrie, J. C.; Strickland, T. W.; Lane, J.; Aoki, K.; Cohen, A. M.; Smalling, R.; Trail, G.; Lin, F. K.; Browne, J. K.; Hines, D. K.: Characterization and biological effects of recombinant human erythropoietin. Immunobiology *172:* 213–224 (1986).

28 Eschbach, J. W.; Adamson, J. W.: Correction of the anemia of hemodialysis (HD) patients with recombinant human erythropoietin (rHuEPO): Results of a multicenter study (Abstract). Kidney int. *33:* 189 (1988).

J. W. Eschbach, MD, Division of Hematology, Department of Medicine, University of Washington, Seattle, WA 98185 (USA)

Discussion

Schaefer (Würzburg): You mentioned that you have experience with 9 predialysis patients. Did you observe an aggravation of hypertension in these patients with EPO treatment?

Eschbach: All of the 9 patients required antihypertensive medication at the beginning and 3 required an increase and adjustment of medication.

Kühn: How does the corrected reticulocyte count in uraemic patients relate to that of normal persons? Is it equal? What would the value be?

Eschbach: The reticulocyte count, corrected for the hematocrit, is about 1%, similar to 'normal' levels. However, we must remember that 'normal' reticulocyte counts and 'normal' serum erythropoietin levels in patients with chronic renal failure are not normal. That is, these values are not what they should be if renal function were normal and anemia of a similar magnitude was present. In such circumstances, the reticulocyte and erythropoietin levels would be 3–10 times greater than 'normal'.

Koch: I was wondering about your comparison between the response of the predialysis patients and that of the dialysis patients. As I recall, the creatinine levels were 7 and 8 mg% in these predialysis patients. Is that really comparable to a dialysis population?

Eschbach: It appears that the rate of response of anemic, pre-dialysis patients with progressive renal disease and hemodialysis patients to recombinant human erythropoietin is similar, at least in the small number of patients that we have observed. In 1 patient who subsequently required hemodialysis, her dose requirement of rhEPO remained essentially unchanged.

Bommer: Concerning the predialysis patients: You know the problem of low protein diet and hypoperfusion of the glomerulus. What is happening with the residual kidney function in predialysis patients under treatment with EPO?

Eschbach: One could theorize that raising the hematocrit would worsen or improve renal function! Fourty years ago, studies in England suggested that transfusions to anemic patients with progressive renal failure worsened renal function. On the other hand, Dr. Barry Brenner has hypothesized that an increased hematocrit will improve renal function. Based upon our limited observations to date, renal function has not deteriorated any faster than anticipated in the small number of patients we have treated with rhEPO.

Caro: I have seen some of your data presented previously and wonder if you have more data on what happens with patients on treatment who get secondary infections? What happens with their anemia and can that be corrected with increasing doses of erythropoietin? I would like you to further comment on this.

Eschbach: Secondary infections or inflammatory conditions can blunt the effectiveness of rhEPO. Dr. Winearls had a patient with pericarditis who had decreased responsiveness to rhEPO for 6 weeks until the pericarditis resolved. Surgery exerts an inflammatory effect and we have observed a decreased responsiveness to rhEPO for 1–4 weeks after surgery, depending upon whether it was for repair of a vascular access or replacement of a hip joint.

Baldamus: The improvement of the anaemia with start of dialysis was attributed to removal of uremic toxins by dialysis. This clinical observation is still valid but you object to the explanation. What then is your interpretation?

Eschbach: The hematocrit may slowly rise in some patients after starting either hemo- or peritoneal dialysis, although it may be more marked in some (but not all) that begin or switch to CAPD. One is inclined to think that this is due to the removal of so-called uremic inhibitors to erythropoiesis by the more permeable peritoneal membrane. However, not all CAPD or hemodialysis patients are observed to increase their hematocrit with dialysis, so the removal of inhibitors, if operative, only applies to some patients, and that raises other questions. On the other hand, we do know that the severely damaged kidney can produce erythropoietin, based upon studies by Drs. Caro and Erslev, so I think it is possible that a slight increase in EPO production, in the absence of marrow suppression by repetitive transfusion, can occur and be responsible for the increase in hematocrit observed in some patients. The liver may also contribute to an increase in EPO production, but unless the patient is anephric, it is impossble to assess that possibility.

Baldamus: But there are some data available especially from Karl Koch's group showing that patients at the time they start dialysis have the highest erythropoietin levels and with increasing hematocrit and improvement of anemia erythropoietin serum levels go down. This is in conflict with your interpretation. Are there really data showing that EPO is lowest at the time dialysis is started and that it increases thereafter with increasing hematocrit.

Eschbach: I am aware of Dr. Koch's article. I believe his group measured EPO with the fetal liver assay. I wonder if there is data using the RIA?

Bauer: Well, I think there was a recent paper in which it was shown that after peritoneal dialysis the EPO went up.

Eschbach: If I recall, serum EPO levels increased after CAPD was initiated. The issue is whether removal of 'inhibitors' allowed for more renal EPO to be produced or whether EPO is made by peritoneal macrophages that are stimulated by the peritoneal lavage technique, and subsequently absorbed into circulation.

Koch: Just a question concerning the issue of PTH or hyperparathyroidism. You very nicely showed that PTH does not inhibit in your in vitro experiments. Do you concede any significant role to hyperparathyroidism at all regarding the degree of renal anemia.

Eschbach: I think that osteitis fibrosa can interfere with the effectiveness of EPO by decreasing marrow space. We have one patient who received very large amounts of rhEPO (1500 U/kg, 3×/week), but responded sluggishly when compared to others treated with the same dose. She had osteitis fibrosa by chest X-ray, and alkaline phosphatase levels were over 800 U/l.

Contr. Nephrol., vol. 66, pp. 71–84 (Karger, Basel 1988)

Specific Problems of Renal Anemia in Childhood

D. E. Müller-Wiefel[a], P. Scigalla[b]

[a]University Children's Hospital, Division of Pediatric Nephrology, Heidelberg, and [b]Boehringer Mannheim GmbH, Mannheim, FRG

Childhood is characterized by a progressive alteration of body composition which is mainly due to growth. Growth is not only age dependent but also characterized by organ-specific growth curves. Changes of the bone marrow with respect to the distribution of bone, fat and red marrow according to age are given in figure 1. Consecutively, the requirements for calories, water, nutrients and trace elements continuously decrease during childhood (table I).

Renal Anemia – Pathomechanisms

On the basis of these observations it is no wonder that differences between children and adults can also be realized in renal anemia [3]. The regression curve between hemoglobin and serum creatinine levels runs at a lower level in pediatric patients compared to adults although both curves start at about the same level (fig. 2). That means, renal anemia is more severe in children than in adults. This observation is probably due to differences in the basic pathogenetic factors: cellular density of *bone marrow* biopsies which was determined morphometrically and expressed as percentage of total volume investigated, was significantly lower in children on either conservative treatment or hemodialysis compared to adults with chronic renal failure [4]. Those only marginally differed from controls (fig. 3). However, the intestinal and extraintestinal *blood loss* estimated in liters/year by different methods was in the same range in children as in adults with chronic renal failure when related to the standard body surface of adults and amounted to 6.7 and 2.6 liters, respectively (table II) [3, 5].

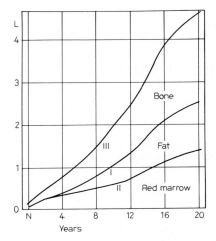

Fig. 1. Anatomy of the bone marrow in childhood [from 1]. N = Neonatal period; L = liters.

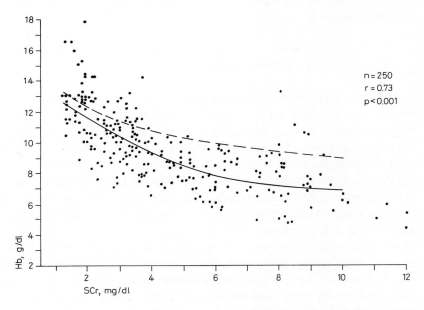

Fig. 2. Correlation between hemoglobin and serum creatinine concentration in children, compared to adults (– – –) [from 3].

Table I. Nutritional requirements in childhood/kg [from 2]

	H₂O, ml	Calories, kcal	Proteins, g	Fe, mg	Folic acid, μg
Infants	150	120	2.0	1.0	50
Small children	100	90	1.5	0.5	20
School children	80	70	1.0	0.4	10
Adolescents	60	50	0.9	0.3	7
Adults	30	30	0.6	0.2	6

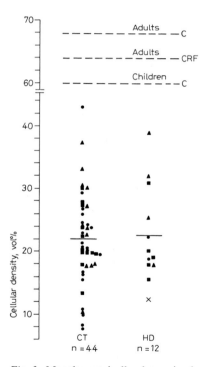

Fig. 3. Morphometrically determined cellular density of bone marrow biopsies expressed as volume percentage (vol%) in uremic children on conservative treatment (CT) and on intermittent hemodialysis (HD), compared to mean values of control (C) children and adults [either controls (C) or with chronic renal failure (CRF)], obtained with the same method [from 3, 5].

Table II. Estimation of blood loss in patients with terminal renal failure [from 3, 5]

Authors	Method	Origin of blood loss		Blood loss l/year
		extraintestinal	intestinal	
Hocken and Marwah	Hb dilution	+	−	1.4–4.6
Mann et al.	Hb dilution	+	−	1.5–3.4
Lindsay and Kennedy	^{51}Cr	+	−	2.0–4.5
Blumberg	^{51}Cr	+	−	1.4–4.0
Koch et al.	^{51}Cr	+	−	2.8
Papadoyanakis et al.	^{51}Cr	−	+	0.9–3.8
Gretz et al.	^{51}Cr	−	+	1.8 ± 1.2
Koch et al.	^{59}Fe	+	+	6.4
Möhring et al.	^{111}In	+	−	2.9
Gretz et al.	^{111}In	−	+	6.8 ± 3.3
Müller-Wiefel[1]	^{111}In	−	+	6.7 ± 1.6
	^{111}In	+	−	2.6 ± 1.6

[1] In children/1.73m² BS.

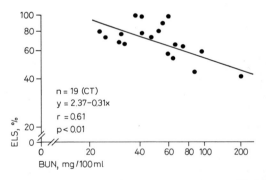

Fig. 4. Inverse correlation between erythrocyte life span (ELS) and blood urea nitrogen (BUN) concentration in children with chronic renal failure [from 3, 4].

Moreover, *erythrocyte life span* which inversely correlated with BUN levels was not found to be decreased to a higher degree than usually observed in adults with renal failure [5]. That means the degree of blood loss and hemolysis does not significantly differ between uremic adults and children (fig. 4).

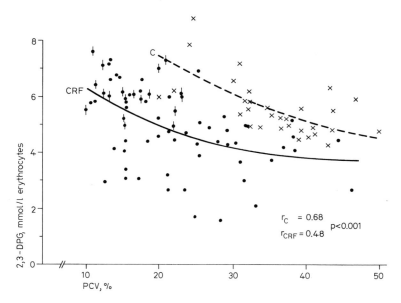

Fig. 5. Inverse correlation between the erythrocyte concentration of 2,3-DPG and packed cell volume (PCV). ● = Children with chronic renal failure; × = children with normal renal function; | = pH >7.45 [from 6].

Hematologic Compensation

Additionally there are major differences in the degree of hematologic compensation of renal anemia between children and grown-ups. Whereas in adults a sufficient increase of *erythrocyte 2,3-DPG* was usually found, the regression curve between this parameter and packed cell volume runs at a lower level in children with renal failure compared to controls [3, 6] (fig. 5).

The inadequate rise of erythrocyte organic phosphates could be ascertained by an insufficient increase of the half saturation pressure of hemoglobin, *p 50,* corrected for a pH of 7.40 (p50c) [7]. Neither on CAPD nor on hemodialysis pressure values reached levels achieved in anemic children without renal failure (fig. 6). That means the hemoglobin oxygen dissociation curve is insufficiently shifted to the right in pediatric patients which is an unusual finding in uremic adults [8].

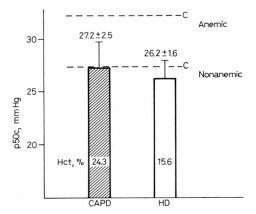

Fig. 6. Mean value of the half saturation pressure of hemoglobin corrected for pH (p50c) in children on CAPD and hemodialysis (HD) compared with anemic controls (C) [from 7].

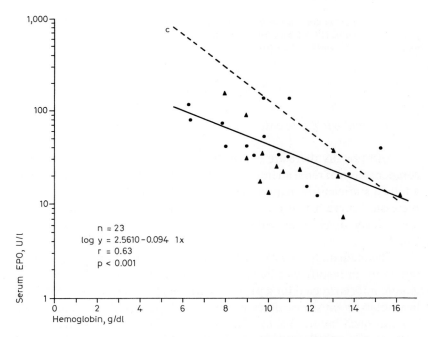

Fig. 7. Inverse linear correlation between serum EPO and hemoglobin, with a minor slope compared to nonuremic control (C) children (n=30) [from 9].

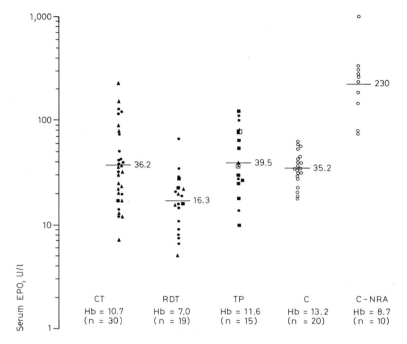

Fig. 8. Variation of EPO concentration in children with chronic renal failure on conservative treatment (CT), regular dialysis treatment (RDT), and after transplatation (TP) compared to normal controls (C) and controls with nonrenal anemia (C-NRA) [from 9].

Erythropoietin (EPO), the indicator of direct hematologic compensation, appears to behave in nearly the same manner as in adults. The hormone increased with decreasing hemoglobin levels. However, the rise was insufficient compared to control children without renal failure [9] (fig. 7). Data were obtained with the fetal mouse liver cell assay system, by which other investigators, however, were not successful in demonstrating a feedback mechanism between EPO secretion and oxygen supply [15]. Whereas a relative EPO deficiency could be detected in children on conservative treatment, an absolute deficiency was found on regular dialysis (fig. 8). Recently the South West Pediatric Nephrologic Study Group – using a radioimmunoassay – was able to demonstrate a clear-cut difference in EPO concentration between children on hemodialysis and those on CAPD which might contribute to the higher hematocrit levels of the latter [10]

Table III. EPO concentrations in children with terminal renal failure [from 10]

	EPO, U/l	Hct, %
HD (n = 41)	24.6 ± 2.1	22.2 ± 0.5
CAPD/CCPD (n = 41)	41.6 ± 5.6*	25.2 ± 0.8**

* p = 0.007; ** p = 0.010.

Table IV. Severity of renal anemia according to puberty of children on RDT [from 11]

	Prepubertal (n = 67)		Pubertal (n = 92)
Hb, g/dl	6.4 ± 1.0	NS	7.2 ± 1.9
Not transfused	17%	p < 0.05	35%

(table III). It has to be elucidated whether EPO plays a role in the severity of renal anemia according to *puberty* of children on regular dialysis treatment. Some years ago already, data of the European Dialysis and Transplant Association demonstrated a significantly lower percentage of nontransfused prepubertal children than of pubertal patients [11] (table IV). This observation might probably be the result of the higher androgenic and consequently higher erythropoietic plasma activity of the pubertal individuals. No difference between adults and children seems to be present concerning the pathogenetic role of hyperparathyroidism in renal anemia [14]. The role of inhibitors of erythropoiesis remains questionable in pediatric patients with uremia, too [16].

Consequences

The consequences of renal anemia affect the cardiovascular system. In uremic children a progressive decrease of the *physical working capacity* could be measured which correlated more intensively with the hemoglobin than with the serum creatinine level [8]. Further direct consequences of renal anemia are decreased well-being, reduced peripheral resistance, uremic heart disease and probably growth failure [14].

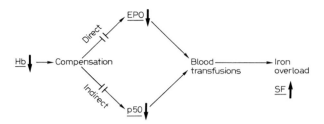

Fig. 9. Mechanism of anemia in children with terminal renal failure leading to iron overload. SF = Serum ferritin.

Table V. Iron load in children with renal failure

	Deficiency (SF < 30 µg/l)	Severe overload (SF > 2,000 µg/l)
Conservative treatment (n = 46)	50%	0%
Hemodialysis (n = 35)	14%	25%
Transplantation (n = 20)	25%	5%

In summary, the anemia of children with terminal renal failure is characterized by an insufficient direct and indirect compensation, that means low EPO and low p50 levels both leading to the need of blood transfusions with the main consequence – *iron overload* (fig. 9). Dependency on blood transfusions is especially typical for children on hemodialysis [12]. During the first year of treatment there is a significant increase of serum ferritin concentrations from 145 to 580 µg/l leading to a progressive iron overload especially of the liver but also of other organ systems such as heart, endocrine glands and bone (fig. 10a–c). On the whole we observed a severe iron overload in 25% of children on hemodialysis but none on conservative treatment, in which half of the patients suffered from iron deficiency (table V). Up to now, iron overload had to be treated with deferoxamine, a potentially hazardous drug. Fortunately, iron overload is less severe in children on CAPD. The reason for this observation is the lower transfusion rate under this mode of treatment (fig. 11). Nevertheless, under CAPD too, iron overload, as measured by the serum ferritin concentration, correlated

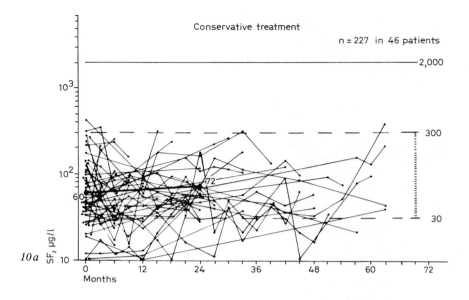

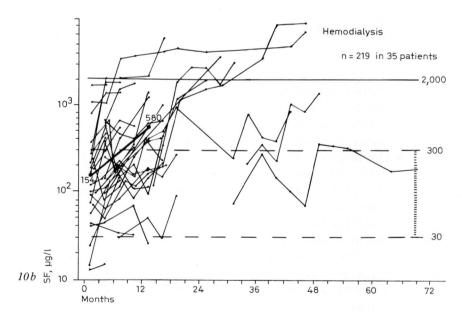

Fig. 10. Course of serum ferritin levels in children with renal failure on conservative treatment *(a)*, on hemodialysis *(b)* and after transplantation *(c)*.

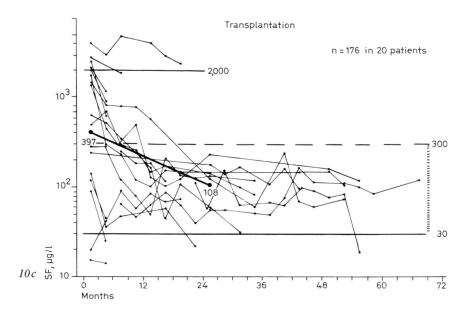

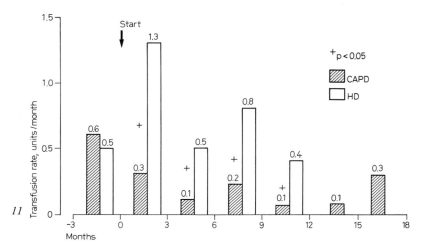

Fig. 11. Transfusion rate in children on hemodialysis and peritoneal dialysis [from 13].

Table VI. Frequency of cytotoxic AB (> 50%) in patients registered for TPL in Heidelberg, 1987

	Patients' age	
	< 20 years	≥ 20 years
Patients, n	24	507
Frequency, %	25	7

$p < 0.05$

with the number of blood transfusions as is the case on hemodialysis [13].

Another negative effect of blood transfusions is the development of *cytotoxic antibodies.* Indeed, the frequency of sensitized patients registered for transplantation in Heidelberg indicated a higher proportion of patients younger than 20 years than of those older than 20 years (table VI). That means a quarter of the children had antibody titers above 50% as the consequence of the higher transfusion rate during this period of life.

The frequency of the third main consequence of a high transfusion rate – namely the *transmission of infective agents,* especially viruses (non-A-non-B-HV, HIV, CMV) – cannot be precisely estimated up to now, but we have the impression that the frequency of this side effect correlates with the number of blood transfusions, too.

The future *therapeutic use of EPO* promises to prevent these side effects of blood transfusions, and could be very beneficial, especially for children with terminal renal failure. We would like to mention in this context that we have started to run a multicenter study for EPO treatment in multiple transfused children and those with iron overload, in which we will carefully watch *body growth.* First experimental data in uremic rats did not give evidence of better growth in EPO-treated uremic animals compared to ad libitum fed controls [17]. However, these uremic animals did not suffer from iron overload so that a clinical effect of EPO on growth in uremic children might nevertheless be expected. The first patient of our study is presented in this issue [18] and we hope that this is a representative example for all children who will profit from EPO treatment in the future.

References

1 Keysserling, K. D. Graf von: Anatomie des Knochenmarks; in Queisser, Das Knochenmark. Morphologie, Funktion, Diagnostik (Thieme, Stuttgart 1978).
2 Deutsche Gesellschaft für Ernährung: Empfehlungen für die Nährstoffzufuhr (Umschauverlag, Frankfurt/Main 1985).
3 Müller-Wiefel, D. E.: Renale Anämie im Kindesalter – Untersuchungen zur Pathogenese und Kompensation (Thieme, Stuttgart 1982).
4 Schärer, K.; Müller-Wiefel, D. E.: Renal anemia in children. A review. Int. J. pediat. Nephrol. *3:* 193–198 (1982).
5 Müller-Wiefel, D. E.; Sinn, H.; Gilli, G.; Schärer, K.: Hemolysis and blood loss in children with chronic renal failure. Clin. Nephrol. *8:* 581–586 (1977).
6 Müller-Wiefel, D. E.; Schärer, K.; Fischer, W.; Michalk, D.: Erythrocyte organic phosphates in the anemia of renal failure in childhood. Eur. J. Pediat. *128:* 103–111 (1978).
7 Müller-Wiefel, D. E.; Bonzel, K. E.; Ruder, H.: Erythrocyte organic phosphates in children on CAPD compared to hemodialysis (HD). Perit. Dial. Bull. *7:* suppl., p. 56 (1987).
8 Schärer, K.; Müller-Wiefel, D. E.: Hemotological problems in renal insufficiency; in Holliday, Barratt, Vernier, Pediatric Nephrology, pp. 880–887 (Williams & Wilkins, Baltimore 1987).
9 Müller-Wiefel, D. E.; Schärer, K.: Serum erythropoietin in children with chronic renal failure. Kidney int. *15:* suppl., pp. 70–76 (1983).
10 Beckmann, B. S.; Brookins, J. W.; Shadduck, R. K.; Mangan, K. F.; Deftos, L. D.; Fisher, J. W.: Effect of different modes of dialysis on serum erythopoeitin levels in children. A report of the Southwest Pediatric Nephrology Study Group. Pediat. Nephrol. (in press).
11 Donckerwolcke, R. A.; Chantler, C.; Broyer, M.; Brunner, F. P.; Brynger, H.; Jacobs, C.; Kramer, P.; Selwood, N. H.; Wing, A. J.: Combined report on regular dialysis and transplantation of children in Europe, 1979; in Robinson, Hawkins, Proceedings of the European Dialysis and Transplant Association, vol. 17, pp. 87–115 (Pitman Medical, London 1980).
12 Müller-Wiefel, D. E.; Waldherr, R.; Feist, B.; v. Kaick, G.: The assessment of iron stores in children on regular dialysis treatment. Contr. Nephrol. vol. 38, pp. 141–152 (Karger, Basel 1984).
13 Müller-Wiefel, D. E.; Bonzel, K. E.; Wartha, R.; Mehls, O.; Schärer, K.: Renal anemia in children on CAPD; in Fine, Schärer, Mehls, CAPD in children, pp. 150–157 (Springer, Berlin 1985).
14 Müller-Wiefel, D. E.; Mehls, O.; Schärer, K.: The role of hyperparathyroidism in the pathogenesis of renal anemia. Eur. J. Pediat. *141:* 63 (1983).
15 Aikhionbare, H. A.; Winterborn, M. W.; Gyde, O. H.: Erythropoietin in children with chronic renal failure on dialytic and nondialytic therapy. Int. J. pediat. Nephrol. *8:* 9–14 (1987)
16 McGonigle, R. J. S.; Boineau, F. G.; Beckman, B.; Ohene-Frempong, K.; Lewy, J. E.; Shadduck, R. K.; Fisher, J. W.: Erythropoietin and inhibitors of in vitro erythropoiesis in the development of anemia in children with renal disease. J. Lab. clin. Med. *105:* 449–458 (1985).

17 Müller-Wiefel, D. E.; Mehls, O.; Schwehm, P.; Gretz, N.; Scigalla, P.: Correction of renal anemia by recombinant human erythropoietin does not improve growth in experimental uremia. Nephrol. Dial. Transplant 2: 399 (1987).

18 Burghard, R.; Leititis, J.; Pallacks, R.; Scigalla, P.; Brandis, M.: Treatment of a seven-year-old child with end-stage renal disease and hemosiderosis by recombinant human erythropoietin. Contr. Nephrol., vol. 66, pp. 139–148 (Karger, Basel 1988).

Priv.-Doz. Dr. Dirk E. Müller-Wiefel, University Children's Hospital,
Im Neuenheimer Feld 150, D-6900 Heidelberg (FRG)

Discussion

Varet: Maybe it is too simple an explanation but when you are a child you have to increase your red cell mass together with your size. Have you looked at the correlation between the increasing weight and height and the degree of anaemia? Because it is interesting to see that after puberty there is no difference to adults. In other words, when you are an adult, you have to maintain your haemoglobin level, but your red cell mass is stable. But when you are a child your red cell mass has to increase every day.

Müller-Wiefel: I would agree, when a child is growing every day. But as you know children, especially with chronic progressive renal failure, have a considerable delay of body growth. So conditions may be rather stable, at least within a period of days and weeks, and the increase of the erythron may be negligible.

Koch: One question concerning your animal experiment: What was the response of these uremic animals regarding hematocrit when you gave erythropoietin?

Müller-Wiefel: Renal anemia could be totally corrected by erythropoietin and we administered erythropoietin in a dosage of 4 units subcutaneously per day. The degree of renal failure was determined by a urea level of around 150 mg/dl.

Koch: And what was the degree of anemia of the uremic control rat?

Müller-Wiefel: I do not have all the data of our experimental study in my mind. If you like, I can show you the slides, but for sure the difference was statistically significant.

Bauer: One hormone that you certainly have considered is the IGF-1, the insulin-like growth factor, because this stimulates both growth and red cell mass. As far as I know, IGF-1 is lower in uremia.

Müller-Wiefel: Yes, it is right. It is part of the determinations in our multicenter study in children. So we will probably get some more information about this phenomenon.

Eschbach: I am interested in the difference between your CAPD and your hemodialysis patients. You showed that in CAPD patients the hematocrit is a little bit higher and that they require less transfusions. Was there any difference in growth rates between children treated with CAPD or hemodialysis?

Müller-Wiefel: No, we did not find any differences in growth rates up to now.

Multicenter Trial of Recombinant Human Erythropoietin: General Results

Contr. Nephrol., vol. 66, pp. 85–93 (Karger, Basel 1988)

Dose-Related Effects of Recombinant Human Erythropoietin on Erythropoiesis

Results of a Multicenter Trial in Patients with
End-Stage Renal Disease

J. Bommer[a], *M. Kugel*[a], *W. Schoeppe*[b], *R. Brunkhorst*[c],
W. Samtleben[d], *P. Bramsiepe*[e], *P. Scigalla*[f]

[a]Medical Clinic, University of Heidelberg; [b]Department of Internal Medicine,
Johann Wolfgang Goethe Universität Frankfurt, Frankfurt/Main; [c]Nephrology
Division, Department of Internal Medicine, Medizinische Hochschule Hannover;
[d]Nephrology Division, Medical Clinic I, Klinikum München-Grosshadern,
Ludwig-Maximilians-Universität, München; [e]Medical Clinic, University of
Cologne; [f]Boehringer Mannheim GmbH, Mannheim, FRG

Inappropriately low serum erythropoietin levels seem to be the major cause of anemia in chronically hemodialyzed patients. In recent publications, several authors described an increase of hematocrit under treatment with recombinant human erythropoietin (rhEPO) [1–4]. After such encouraging initial results, careful studies to delineate optimal dose and most effective frequency of rhEPO application are required. Furthermore, more in-depth analysis of potential side effects is desirable. In the following, we report on a randomized multicenter study of 95 patients from 5 German University Hospitals which was designed to address these points.

Material and Methods

Patients

Ninety-five patients initially entered the study to be treated with rhEPO (Boehringer Co., Mannheim, FRG).

In 52 patients, uremia resulted from glomerular diseases like glomerulonephritis, diabetes, amyloidosis, in 34 patients from a non-glomerular disease like nephrolithiasis, malformation, polycystic kidney disease, analgesic abuse, nephrocalcinosis, interstitial nephritis, etc. In 9 patients, the underlying disease was not known. None of the patients had received immunosuppressive therapy during the last 3 months before rhEPO treatment.

Table I. Baseline data collected during the run-in period in patients treated with 40, 80 or 120 U (G 40, G 80, G 120) rhEPO/kg body weight 3 ×/week

	G 40	G 80	G 120
Number of patients	31	29	28
Age	51 (21–67)	52 (22–74)	41 (21–74)
Duration of dialysis, months	68 (6–172)	60 (6–181)	50 (6–146)
Hematocrit, %	22.3 (16–28)	22.1 (15.6–27.3)	21.4 (16–27)
MCHC, g/dl	33.4 (31–37)	32.9 (30–34)	33.5 (30–35)
Corrected reticulocyte, %	0.68 (0.3–2.1)	0.71 (0.3–2.0)	0.64 (0.2–1.7)

Ranges are shown in parentheses.

Symptoms or clinical findings of vitamin B_{12} and folic acid deficiency, intoxication by aluminum, hemolysis, gastrointestinal bleeding or severe hyperparathyroidism were not observed in the patients.

In the study, such patients were included, who fulfilled the following criteria: hematocrit <28%, age >18 years, duration of hemodialysis >6 months, no transfusions.

Study Protocol

It was the aim of the study to raise serum hematocrit levels of anemic dialysis patients by at least 10% into the range of 30–35% or to an absolute value of at least 35% if the baseline values were 25–28%. After a run-in period of 2 weeks in which baseline date were collected, patients were divided randomly into 3 groups. As shown in table I, baseline data of patients available for study of efficacy were comparable in all 3 groups. The median age of patients receiving 120 U rhEPO/kg body weight was somewhat lower compared to the other groups, but the difference was not significant. During the dose-finding or correction period, patients received three times weekly either 40 U rhEPO per kg body weight (group 40) or 80 U rhEPO/kg body weight (group 80) or 120 U rhEPO/kg body weight (group 120). If the hematocrit of patients did not reach target levels of 30–35% after 12 weeks, the rhEPO dose was increased from 40 to 80 or from 80 to 120 U rhEPO/kg, respectively, depending on the initial dose. If in patients of group 40 the increase of rhEPO to 80 U did not raise hematocrit to the target level during the following 4 weeks, the rhEPO dose was further increased to 120 U rhEPO/kg thrice weekly.

If hematocrit levels had risen to 30–35%, an effort was made to reduce the rhEPO dose so that hematocrit was maintained at a constant level. It has been intended to treat all patients with the same protocol during the follow-up period. However, the protocol was violated by one of the five centers. Consequently, separate data will be presented for a patient cohort treated according to the pre-arranged protocol (three times per week 15 U/kg rhEPO or more, if higher dose was necessary) and one patient cohort in which the dose of the dose finding period (40, 80 or 120 U per injection) was left unchanged, but frequency of administration reduced to twice or once per week.

Laboratory Measurements

Hematological profile (Coulter counter) was measured before each dialysis three times weekly. Blood chemistry was determined once a week (multichannel autoanalyser). Ferritin (radioimmunoassay), transferrin (immunodiffusion) and haptoglobin (laser nephelometry) were controlled monthly. Reticulocyte counts were either corrected for anemia or expressed as absolute reticulocyte counts.

Statistical Analysis

For a comparison of the three independent groups with respect to the target parameter of the study – the average weekly increase in hematocrit – a sample calculation was included in the study plan in order to be able to test for differences between the group in a conformatory sense during evaluation with a multiple level of significance of 5% and a power of 95%.

The distribution-free rank sum test by Wilcoxon was used as part of the closed multiple testing procedure [10, 11]. Medians, interquartile ranges and extreme values were determined as appropriate position and distribution parameters.

During the course of the study, 12 patients received a kidney transplant. In 8 patients, rhEPO treatment was discontinued for various reasons (hypertensive crises: 4 patients; cardiovascular complications: 1 patient; subdural hematoma: 1 patient; 2 patients refused to continue the study). Four patients reentered the study after an rhEPO-free period of several weeks. Data for statistical evaluation were available from 92 of the originally 95 patients. All 92 patients were evaluated with regard to safety and tolerance. Four of the 92 patients could not be included in the evaluation for efficacy because the duration of therapy was too short (<2 weeks in 3 patients) or the application frequency differed (1 patient). Thus, for the correction phase, data of only 88 patients were available for the evaluation for efficacy (see table II). Eighty-five of these 88 patients were treated for 12 weeks or more. At the time evaluation (October 1987, 18–28 weeks after onset of EPO therapy), laboratory data from the maintenance period were available of only 62 patients, since in particular the patients receiving 40 U/kg body weight had not yet reached the target hematocrit (see table II). For graphical analysis the number of patients was further reduced to 51 since only those patients were included who had been in the maintenance period for a minimum of 5 weeks (see fig. 3, 4).

At the present time (November 1987) 79 patients are still being treated with rhEPO as part of this study (24–34 weeks, average 30 weeks). Two of these patients have not yet reached the target hematocrit, 4 patients were admitted again into the study after unsuccessful kidney transplantation and must be analyzed separately. Seventy-three patients are in the maintenance period and receive different rhEPO doses (see table III).

Results

In the second week of rhEPO treatment, hematocrit started to increase in patients of group 80 and 120 (fig. 1). In patients of group 40, hematocrit levels increased 1 week later during the third week. The median percent increment of hematocrit per week during the dose-finding period was 0.69%

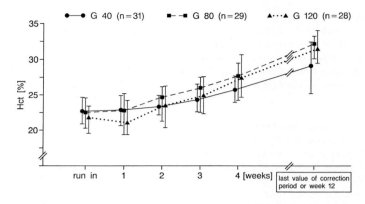

Fig. 1. Median hematocrit levels during rhEPO therapy (dose-finding period).

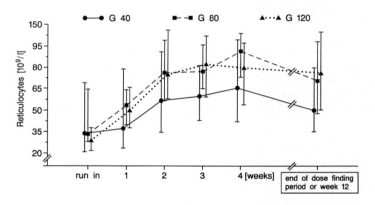

Fig. 2. Median of absolute reticulocyte counts under rhEPO therapy during the dose-finding period. G 40: n = 31; G 80: n = 29; G 120: n = 28.

in group 40, 1.25% in group 80 and 1.55% in group 120, i.e. the increment was dose dependent and statistically significant between group 40 and group 80 as well as between group 40 and group 120 (p<0.05).

Reticulocyte counts increased during the first week with the protocol administering three times weekly 80 or 120 U/kg rhEPO (fig. 2). In patients of group 40, reticulocyte counts did not increase before the second week of rhEPO treatment. After 3–4 weeks, reticulocyte counts reached a maximum

Table II. Hematological findings in patients during the run-in period as well as during the dose-finding period and long-term follow-up period of rhEPO therapy

	Run-in period		Last value of correction period or week 12		Last value in maintenance period	
Erythrocytes, 10^{12}/l	2.30 (1.13–3.42)	$\left.\right\}$ n = 88	3.20 (1.3–4.3)	$\left.\right\}$ n = 88	3.20 (1.70–4.28)	$\left.\right\}$ n =62
MCV, μm^3	95.9 (82–144)		96.4 (76–146)		94.5 (84–115)	
MCHC, g/dl	33.3 (29.7–37.0)		32.1 (25.4–40.3)		32.8 (28.8–35.7)	
Leukocytes, 10^9/l	6.82 (3.40–14.53)	$\left.\right\}$ n = 92	6.90 (3.05–15.7)	$\left.\right\}$ n = 92	7.10 (3.0–11.7)	$\left.\right\}$ n = 62
Neutrophils, %	63.3 (38–78)		64 (21–86)		62 (32–80)	
Eosinophils, %	3.7 (0–23.7)		4 (0–26.0)		3 (0–37.0)	
Lymphocytes, %	26.8 (13.3–47.7)		26 (8–53)		25.5 (12–50.0)	
Monocytes, %	4.0 (0.5–8.7)		4.0 (0–14.0)		4.0 (0–11.0)	
Platelets, 10^9/l	229 (67–568)		260 (70–650)		243 (73–456)	

Ranges shown in parentheses.

in all groups. The maximal level of reticulocyte counts was not different in patients of groups 80 and 120, but was significantly lower in group 40 ($p < 0.05$).

As shown in table II, no change of mean corpuscular volume (MCV) and mean corpuscular hemoglobin concentration (MCHC), granulocytes or differential blood count was noted during the study period. Platelet number increased during rhEPO therapy; this will be discussed in detail in the paper by Grützmacher et al. in this volume [8].

The primarily unintended differences in dosage strategies during the maintenance phase of the study necessitated separate evaluation of the data collected during the maintenance period. In 4 of 5 centers, where the patients received 3 times per week 15 U rhEPO/kg body weight or more if necessary, hematocrit remained unchanged until the 4th week and decreased subsequently (fig. 3). Reticulocytes decreased during the first 4 weeks and increased when the dose of rhEPO was raised subsequently (fig. 4). In contrast, in the cohort of patients receiving 1 or 2 administrations of rhEPO per week, without reduction of the dose per injection which had been administered during the dose-finding period, hematocrit remained unchanged but reticulocyte counts decreased (fig. 3, 4).

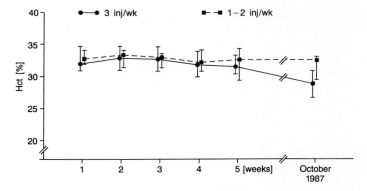

Fig. 3. Median hematocrit levels under rhEPO therapy during the long-term follow-up study period. October 1987 = 18–28 weeks after start of rhEPO therapy.

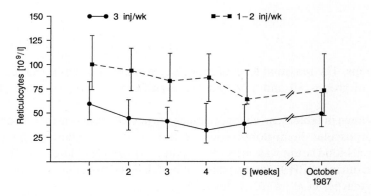

Fig. 4. Median of absolute reticulocyte counts under rhEPO therapy during the long-term follow-up study period. October 1987 = 18–28 weeks after start of rhEPO therapy.

Post hoc analysis in November 1987 in 73 patients showed, however, that the weekly dose of rhEPO required to maintain the target hematocrit level was higher for patients with 1–2 administrations per week (median 160 U/kg per week, range 40–240) than for patients with 3 administrations per week (median 90 U/kg per week, range 22–240) (table III).

Table III. Number of patients requiring different maintenance doses of rhEPO (November 1987, 24–34 weeks after start of rhEPO therapy)

	Maintenance dose of rhEPO/week				
	< 60	80–90	120–155	160–180	225–240
1–2 ×/week	1	3	2	6	5
3 ×/week	14	21	11	6	4

The total rhEPO dose per week was lower in patients receiving three injections per week compared to patients given only 1–2 injections per week.

Discussion

In our randomized multicenter study, we confirm the observation that rhEPO induces a dose-dependent increase of reticulocyte counts and hematocrit levels in anemic dialysis patients [1–7]. The increment of reticulocytes was greater in patients receiving three times per week 80 and 120 U rhEPO /kg body weight compared to patients receiving only 40 U rhEPO/kg body weight. Correspondingly, the median increment of hematocrit per week was significantly higher in group 80 and group 120 than in group 40. The increment appeared to be dose-dependent, however, the difference between group 80 and group 120 (1.25 versus 1.55%) was statistically not significant.

During the maintenance period, reduction of rhEPO dose or of the frequency of application of rhEPO was followed by an initial decrease of hematocrit and/or absolute reticulocyte count. These changes in the two populations with different therapy strategies obviously were due to difficulties in establishing the adequate rhEPO maintenance dose or frequency of application, as post hoc analysis showed a return to target hematocrit in all patients. The observation that less rhEPO (U per week) was necessary to maintain the target hematocrit, when rhEPO was given in three injections per week, compared to 1–2 injections per week, may point to an increased efficacy of rhEPO when administrations are spaced at shorter intervals. Since the more physiological mode of administration would be continuous rhEPO infusion, an alternate mode of more frequent administration should be explored.

References

1 Winearls, C.G.; Oliver, D.; Pippard, M.J.; Reid, C.; Downing, M.R.; Cotes, P.M.: Effect of human erythropoietin derived from recombinant DNA on the anemia of patients maintained by chronic hemodialysis. Lancet *ii:* 1175–1178 (1986).

2 Eschbach, J.W.; Egrie, J.C.; Downing, M.R.; Browne, J.K.; Adamson, J.W.: Correction of the anemia of end-stage renal disease with recombinant human erythropoietin. New Engl. J. Med. *316:* 73–78 (1987).

3 Bommer, J.; Alexiou, C.; Müller-Bühl, E.; Eifert, J.; Ritz, E.: Recombinant human erythropoietin therapy in haemodialysis patients – dose determination and clinical experience. Nephrol. Dial. Transplant. *2:* 238–242 (1987).

4 Zins, B.; Drüeke, T.; Zinpratt, J.; et al.: Erythropoietin treatment in anemic patients on hemodialysis. Lancet *ii:* 1329 (1986).

5 Bommer, J.; Müller-Bühl, E.; Ritz, E.; Eifert, J.: Recombinant human erythropoietin in anaemic patients on haemodialysis (Letter). Lancet *i:* 392 (1987).

6 Casati, S.; Passerini, P.; Campise, M.R.; Graziani, G.; Cesana, B.; Perisic, M.; Ponticelli, C.: Benefits and risks of protracted treatment with human recombinant erythropoietin in patients having haemodialyis. Br. med. J. *295:* 1017–1020 (1987).

7 Stutz, B.; Rhyner, K.; Vögtli, J.; Binswanger, U.: Erfolgreiche Behandlung der Anämie bei Hämodialyse-Patienten mit rekombiniertem humanem Erythropoietin. Schweiz. med. Wschr. *117:* 1397–1402 (1987).

8 Grützmacher, P.; Bergmann, M.; Weinreich, T.; Nattermann, U.; Reimers, E.; Pollok, M.: Beneficial and adverse effects of correction of anaemia by recombinant human erythropoietin in patients on maintenance haemodialysis. Contr. Nephrol., vol. 66, pp. 104–113 (Karger, Basel 1988).

9 Kühn, K.; Nonnast-Daniel, B.; Grützmacher, P.; Grüner, J.; Pfäffl, W.; Baldamus, C.A.; Scigalla, P.: Analysis of initial resistance of erythropoiesis to treatment with recombinant human erythopoietin. Contr. Nephrol., vol. 66, pp. 94–103 (Karger, Basel 1988).

10 Hollander, M.; Wolfe, D.: Nonparametric statistical methods, p. 26ff. (J. Wiley & Sons, New York 1973).

11 Einot, I.; Gabriel, K.R.: A study of power of several methods of multiple comparison. J. Am. Statist. Ass. *7:* 574 (1975).

Prof. Dr. Jürgen Bommer, Medical Clinic, University of Heidelberg, Bergheimer Strasse 58, D–6900 Heidelberg (FRG)

Discussion

Klinkmann (Rostock): Dr. Bommer, we are now coming to the clinical applications. I was impressed by your rather high number of drop-outs. Could you just give us certain explanations?

Bommer: I have detailed information, but I think it will be the topic of the following speakers, so I would like to give these questions and the problems to my following speakers.

Eschbach: I am interested in the feasibility of giving rhEPO on a weekly rather than a triweekly basis, due to the fact that the pharmacokinetics indicate that rhEPO has a relatively short half-life of 6–9 h. Do you have any explanation as to how you can get by with a longer duration between doses? In one slide differences in the other centers were noted. These other centers suggest there was a drop of the hematocrit from about 33 to 29 when dosing on a weekly basis. Was that a significant drop?

Bommer: Concerning the half-life of EPO: as we discussed in the morning, the half-life of recombinant human EPO is about 4.8 h and at the EDTA in London, Dr. Winearls has shown a very impressive slide indicating that after 12 or 14 h, rhEPO is no more effective due to the short half-life time or cellular sequestration of the EPO.

I can only report the data obtained in different centers; I cannot speculate what would be the optimal or the minimal dose of rhEPO we need, if the EPO was given by continuous infusion or given by twice daily injections or so. I expect under these conditions the EPO dose would be much less than the dose used at the moment. Presently, we are using pharmacological doses of rhEPO given as pulse stimulation and not as a physiological continuous stimulation.

Concerning the reduction of the hematocrit levels: As you know, we had experience obtained in a previous study. In that study, we observed a continuous rise of hematocrit during the following weeks even if the rhEPO dose was reduced; therefore, in this study, we reduced the rhEPO dose in our patients rather early, but we decreased in our patients perhaps the dose of EPO a little bit less than was done in the other units. In these other units, a more severe reduction was followed by a decrease of hematocrit levels after 4 weeks. When you consider that the hematocrit levels continue to increase for 2 weeks when the rh EPO dose is reduced, a time lag of 4 weeks was to be expected until the hematocrit levels decreased when the EPO dose was reduced too intensively. That would explain the drop of hematocrit in the 4 other centers 4 weeks after reduction of rhEPO.

In these patients receiving a very low rhEPO dose during the first weeks of the follow-up period, reticulocyte counts increased at the end of the observation period. This was due to a higher rhEPO dose during the last weeks of the observation period. During the following week, a rise of hematocrit has to be expected, too.

Bauer: I wonder why you fixed a target hematocrit for which you were shooting rather than a physiological measure, like heart rate at a work load or something like this, because the hematocrit of 30 may mean different things in different patients.

Bommer: At the moment, we are all looking for the best or the optimal hematocrit levels required in our patients. You know the complications resulting from a very steep rise of hematocrit observed in the study of Eschbach and Winearls. They observed some hypertensive crises and other problems which are under discussion. The factors and mechanisms underlying these complications are not clarified.

In our opinion, the increasing viscosity, particularly the rapid change of the viscosity of blood, is one important factor, favouring a hypertensive blood pressure. I think these problems will be discussed in the following presentation.

At the moment, we do not know whether hematocrit levels of 30 or 35 are the optimum for our patients. In our patients, we realised that physical activity and well-being was not better in patients when hematocrit levels were >35% under EPO treatment. In this respect, fistula clotting must be considered. We have the feeling that fistual clotting is more frequent if hematocrit levels increase under EPO treatment. I think a hematocrit level of 30% is, at the moment, a compromise.

Contr. Nephrol., vol. 66, pp. 94–103 (Karger, Basel 1988)

Analysis of Initial Resistance of Erythropoiesis to Treatment with Recombinant Human Erythropoietin

Results of a Multicenter Trial in Patients with End-Stage Renal Disease

K. Kühn[a], *B. Nonnast-Daniel*[a], *P. Grützmacher*[b], *J. Grüner*[c], *W. Pfäffl*[d], *C. A. Baldamus*[e], *P. Scigalla*[f]

[a]Medizinische Hochschule Hannover; Medizinische Kliniken der Universitäten [b]Frankfurt/M., [c]Heidelberg, [d]München, [e]Köln, und [f]Boehringer Mannheim, Mannheim, BRD

In preceding trials of human recombinant erythropoietin (rhEPO) in the treatment of renal anemia it became evident that the response of patients with end-stage renal disease may be variable even when equal doses were applied [2, 4, 6]. In the present study we analyzed the incidence of initial total or partial resistance to rhEPO and also factors possibly responsible for the variable response in patients participating in a multicenter trial.

Methods

According to the protocol of the study [1], patients received either 40, 80 or 120 IU/kg rhEPO 3 times/week at the end of the hemodialysis for a planned period of 12 weeks. When hematocrit (HCT) had increased by 10 vol% and above an absolute value of 30 vol% or less than 10 vol% but above an absolute value of 35 vol% before or at the end of the 12-week treatment period, patients were switched to a maintenance dose sufficient to keep the HCTs at the achieved levels. Those patients who did not reach the above stated end points within 12 weeks were switched to higher doses. Once they fulfilled end-point criteria they were also switched to maintenance doses.

Values of reticulocytes were corrected for the degree of anemia as described by Ganzoni [5]. The majority of the patients had an oral iron supplementation (equivalent of 200 mg Fe^{++}/day). Serum ferritin was regularly monitored. When serum ferritin levels decreased to 60 ng/l, iron was supplemented intravenously to replenish iron stores. *Initial nonresponse* was defined as no increase of HCT within 12 weeks of treatment using the

Table I. Patients with initial nonresponse or initially reduced response to rhEPO treatment

rhEPO dose, IU/kg (3 times/week)	N	NR	RR
120	28	–	2
80	28	1	2
40	29	4	17

N = Number of analyzed patients; NR = number of patients with nonresponse; RR = number of patients with reduced response.

same rhEPO dose. *Initially reduced response* was assumed when HCT increased by less than 10 vol% within 12 weeks of treatment using the same rhEPO dose. Not categorized as reduced responders were those patients whose HCT had risen above 35 vol% although the increase was less than 10 vol%.

Results

Among 85 rhEPO-treated patients analyzed, 5 did not respond with an increase of HCT after a treatment period of 12 weeks. Four of these patients received 40 IU/kg, 1 of them 80 IU/kg rhEPO (table I). Seventeen out of 29 patients who received 40 IU/kg rhEPO, 2 out of 28 patients who were treated with 80 IU/kg and 2 out of 28 patients who received 120 IU/kg had a reduced response to rhEPO treatment (table I).

Patients with Initial Nonresponse to rhEPO Therapy

The age of these patients was between 21 and 66 years. Chronic renal failure was caused by cystic kidney disease in 1 patient and by glomerulonephritis in 4 patients. HCT varied between 21 and 28% prior to rhEPO treatment (table II). Further data of these patients are listed in table III.

Patient 118 did not respond to 80 IU/kg rhEPO within the first 12 weeks. There was a moderate decrease of serum ferritin during treatment. Corrected reticulocyte count was high prior and under rhEPO treatment. After 12 weeks of rhEpo-treatment with 80 IU/kg, the rhEPO dose was raised to 120 IU/kg and iron substituted intravenously which resulted in an increase of HCT. The patient had received blood transfusions once per month for at least 1 year prior to rhEPO treatment. Despite these poly-transfusions, the pretreatment serum ferritin level was not high. We attri-

Table II. Initial nonresponders under rhEPO therapy

Patient No.	Age	Renal disease	HCT before treatment, %	rhEPO dose, IU/kg (3 times/week)
118	64	glomerulonephritis	25	80
217	21	glomerulonephritis	22	40
312	51	glomerulonephritis	25	40
409	59	glomerulonephritis	21	40
503	66	cystic kidney disease	28	40

Table III. Initial nonresponders under rhEPO therapy

Patient No.	Ferritin, ng/ml (prior/during rhEPO)	Corrected reti-culocyte counts, % (prior/during rhEPO)	Assumed causes of nonresponse	Effect of change of therapy after 12 weeks
118	110/80	3.0/1.8	increased blood loss	+ (dose ↑, Fe i.v.)
217	85/39	0.6/0.6	iron deficiency	+ (dose ↑, Fe i.v.)
312	65/50	0.8/1.5–0.8	infection during rhEPO therapy	+ (dose ↑, Fe i.v.)
409	320/520	0.5/0.8	no response to erythropoiesis; inadequate rhEPO dose	+ (dose ↑)
503	220/70	0.8/1.3	inadequate rhEPO dose; increased blood loss?	+ (dose ↑)

bute the initial failure of response in this patient to an increased blood loss, presumably also during treatment.

Patient 217 had a low normal pretreatment ferritin level which decreased with rhEPO therapy (40 IU/kg). Corrected reticulocyte count was rather low before and on treatment. Following an increase of rhEPO dose to 80 IU/kg and intravenous iron substitution, the patient's HCT increased. The initial nonresponse was probably due to iron deficiency.

Patient 312 initially responded very well to rhEPO therapy (40 IU/kg). HCT decreased again with further treatment. Serum ferritin prior to therapy was rather low. Corrected reticulocyte count increased initially under rhEPO therapy but later on decreased again. This coincided with an acute infection of the urinary bladder which needed antibiotic treatment. After 12 weeks an increase of rhEPO dose to 80 IU/kg and intravenous iron substitution led to an increase of HCT. We assume that failure to respond in this patient was caused by infection.

Patient 409 was the only among the nonresponders who had a high pretreatment serum ferritin level which remained elevated under rhEPO therapy (40 IU/kg) without iron substitution. Corrected reticulocyte count was low prior to treatment and increased slowly under the initial rhEPO therapy. After 12 weeks an HCT increase was achieved by increasing the rhEPO dose to 80 IU/kg. In this patient the initial rhEPO dose was probably too low to stimulate erythropoiesis.

Patient 503 was polytransfused (9 transfusions in the last 12 months prior to rhEPO therapy). In spite of this, pretreatment serum ferritin was within the normal range and decreased further under therapy. Pretreatment-corrected reticulocyte count was at the lower normal level and increased slightly under therapy. After 12 weeks he responded to a higher rhEPO dose (80 IU/kg). The initial nonresponse seems to be caused by increased blood loss. With regard to a high blood loss, the initial rhEPO dose was probably inadequate.

Patients with Initially Reduced Response to rhEPO Therapy

Seventeen out of 29 patients who received an initial rhEPO dose of 40 IU/kg had a reduced response. All of them reacted with a further rise of HCT when after 12 weeks of initial treatment either the rhEPO dose was raised to 80 IU/kg (8 patients) or iron was substituted intravenously and the rhEPO dose was raised (8 patients) or antibiotic treatment of an infection was performed (1 patient) (table IV). Four out of 56 patients who were treated with 80 or 120 IU/kg rhEPO also had a reduced response within the first 12 weeks of therapy. One patient who was initially treated with 80 IU/kg responded well to a higher rhEPO dose (120 IU/kg). Since he had a normal value of serum ferritin and a normal corrected reticulocyte count prior to and under rhEPO treatment, it was assumed that his reduced increase of HCT was caused by an inadequate initial rhEPO dose (table V). The other 3 patients, 1 of them treated with 80 IU/kg and 2 with 120 IU/kg, responded well to an intravenous iron substitution (table V); in 1 of them treated with 120 IU/kg there was evidence of major intestinal blood loss.

Table IV. Patients with initially reduced response under rhEPO therapy (40 IU/kg 3 times/week)

Patients, n	Assumed causes of reduced response	Effect of change of therapy after 12 weeks
8	inadequate rhEPO dose	+ (rhEPO dose ↑)
8	iron deficiency	+ (Fe i.v., rhEPO dose ↑)
1	infection	+ (antibiotic treatment)

Table V. Patients with initially reduced response under rhEPO therapy

rhEPO dose, IU/kg (3 times/week)	Patients, n	Assumed causes of reduced response	Effect of change of therapy after 12 weeks
80	1	inadequate response to rhEPO dose	+ (rhEPO dose ↑)
80	1	iron deficiency	+ (Fe i.v.)
120	1	intestinal bleeding; iron deficiency	+ (Fe i.v.)
120	1	iron deficiency	+ (Fe i.v.)

Discussion

Our study has demonstrated that in 21 out of 29 patients who received only 40 IU/kg rhEPO, no rise of HCT occurred or the rise was not sufficient following the criteria set by us. In contrast, in patients who were treated with 80 or 120 IU/kg rhEPO, only 3 and 2 respectively out of 28 patients in each group had a reduced or no response. These results confirm the observation of a dose-dependent effect of rhEPO treatment [1, 4].

Analysis of the 5 patients who had *no response* of HCT within 12 weeks of initial rhEPO treatment revealed that 2 of them who were in need of regular polytransfusions prior to rhEPO therapy had probably an increased blood loss; 1 patient had major iron deficiency; 1 had an infection during therapy and 1 patient did not respond to the initial rhEPO dose without

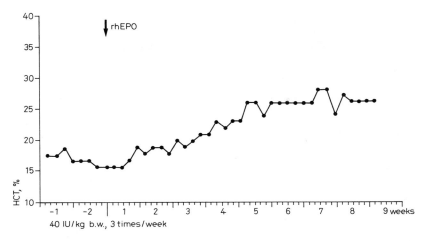

Fig. 1. Typical course of HCT in a patient with initially reduced response to rhEPO treatment.

evidence of other reasons (table III). This last patient (409) was the only among the nonresponders who had a high serum ferritin level before and under treatment. Since this coincided with a low corrected reticulocyte count under 40 IU/kg rhEPO therapy, it is obvious that his rhEPO dose was inadequate.

The main reasons for an *initially reduced response* to rhEPO therapy were an inadequate rhEPO dose and an iron insufficiency (table IV, V). Among patients with an initial partial resistance the course of HCT under therapy was very often characterized by the same pattern (fig. 1). An initial increase was followed by a plateau representing obviously a steady state between erythropoiesis and opposing factors such as reduced erythrocyte life span and blood loss.

Other factors which could account for no or a reduced response were also evaluated in our patients. However, there was no evidence for a severe hyperparathyroidism, major hemolysis, signs of inadequate dialysis or of aluminum intoxication. With regard to the role of aluminum in renal anemia [3], we have not studied in our patients whether there exists a negative correlation between plasma aluminium concentration after desferrioxamine and the response to rhEPO treatment as recently reported by Casati et al. [2].

Additional information regarding the mechanism of no or reduced response to rhEPO treatment can be expected when patients will be switched to rhEPO maintenance doses after finally having reached the treatment goal. Surprisingly, so far there seem to be no significant differences in the mean maintenance doses between all analyzed rhEPO treated patients and those who were nonresponders or reduced responders to initial treatment.

From our studies of initial resistance to rhEPO it can be concluded that among 85 patients evaluated there was no patient who at the end did not respond to rhEPO therapy. Beside the fact that 40 IU/kg was an inadequate rhEPO dose in several patients, the major cause of no or reduced response to rhEPO treatment was iron deficiency. In spite of oral iron supplementation, iron deficiency may occur in a significant percentage of ESRD patients when erythropoiesis improves under rhEPO therapy necessitating intravenous iron supplementation.

References

1   Bommer, J.; Kugel, M.; Schoeppe, W.; Brunkhorst, R.; Samtleben, W.; Bramsiepe, P.: Dose-related effects of recombinant human erythropoietin on erythropoiesis. Results of a multicenter trial in patients with end-stage renal disease. Contr. Nephrol., vol. 66, pp. 85–93 (Karger, Basel 1988).
2   Casati, S.; Passerini, P.; Campise, M. R.; Graziani, G.; Cesana, B.; Perisic, M.; Ponticelli, C.: Benefits and risks of protracted treatment with human recombinant erythropoietin in patients having hemodialysis. Br. med. J. *295:* 1017–1021 (1987).
3   Eschbach, J. W.; Adamson, J. W.: Anemia of end-stage renal disease. Kidney int. *28:* 1–5 (1985).
4   Eschbach, J. W.; Egrie, J. C.; Downing, M. R.; Browne, J. K.; Adamson, J. W.: Correction of anemia of end-stage renal disease (ESRD) with recombinant human erythropoietin: Results of a phase I–II clinical trial. New Engl. J. Med. *316:* 73–78 (1987).
5   Ganzoni, A. M.: Die Bedeutung der Retikulozyten-Zahl für die Beurteilung einer Anämie. Dt. med. Wschr. *59:* 2291–2292 (1970).
6   Winearls, C. G.; Oliver, D. O.; Pippard, M. J.; Reid, C.; Downing, M. R.; Cotes, P. M.: Effect of human erythropoietin derived from recombinant DNA on the anemia of patients maintained by chronic hemodialysis. Lancet *ii:* 1175–1178 (1986).

Prof. Dr. med. K. Kühn, Medizinische Hochschule Hannover,
Zentrum Innere Medizin und Dermatologie, Konstanty-Gutschow-Strasse 8,
D-3000 Hannover 61 (FRG)

Discussion

Müller-Wiefel: Could you tell us what happened to the mean corpuscular volume and the mean corpuscular hemoglobin concentration of the erythrocytes, especially in those patients who responded after iron treatment, and did I understand you correctly that none of your patients suffered from aluminum toxicity and none of your patients suffered from extreme secondary hyperparathyroidism?

Kühn: The answer to the last question is yes. In answer to the first question: we did not yet analyze our data regarding changes of mean corpuscular volume and mean corpuscular hemoglobin concentration following iron substitution.

Bommer: Concerning hyperparathyroidism, I would like to make a comment. In another study of rhEPO response in uremic patients, we had a patient who suffered from acute hyperparathyroidism and had to be parathyroidectomised during the rhEPO treatment. The response to EPO was absolutely normal in this patient when she suffered from acute hyperparathyroidism. We did not find an interaction between clinical hyperparathyroidism and EPO response.

Kühn: There was no patient with severe hyperparathyroidism and severe aluminum intoxication among our nonresponders and reduced responders.

Koch: Dr. Bommer, do you have bone histology of the patient you just described?

Bommer: We have no histology of the bone, but we have X-ray of the skeleton which showed typical bone resorption and spongiosation of the corticalis in the finger. We have a histology of the parathyroid gland. The patient had a high alkaline phosphatase which decreased after parathyroidectomy. The patient was not vitamin D deficient and no marked aluminum intoxication was found using the DFO provocation test.

Klinkmann (Rostock): In the strict meaning of the word, at least in the strict scientific meaning of the word, since you had only dose-dependent nonresponders, you could probably state that there are no real nonresponders at all among your material.

Kühn: That was our conclusion. At the end all patients responded. We had no definite nonresponders.

Klinkmann: My question to the audience is: Did anybody ever observe a real nonresponder at all, not a dose-related nonresponder? As far as the literature is concerned, Dr. Eschbach, do you know anybody who did finally not respond? All nonresponse was dose dependent or infection related, but there is not a single case in my mind who did not finally respond.

Eschbach: We had one patient who was unresponsive and had a low MCV, but was not iron-deficient. She was treated with 300 U/kg rhEPO three times a week, per protocol. After 4 weeks of treatment, she had not responded. We thought she was aluminum overloaded because she had a marked delta in her aluminum level after desferrioxamine challenge. We then treated with desferrioxamine (DFO) for about 6 months. Since the delta aluminum levels after DFO had improved, she was retreated at 150 U/kg, 3 ×/wk, and after another 4 weeks had still not responded. She also has alpha-thalassemia, but alpha-thalassemics are usually not anemic. I am not sure why she did not respond to rhEPO.

Caro: I wonder if anybody has done bone marrow examinations on these patients that have normal or even elevated levels of ferritin and still appear to be iron deficient. Ferritin is an acute and chronic phase-reactant protein, the levels do not necessarily represent bone marrow iron stores and I think that you have to solve the question whether this is a problem of marrow iron reutilisation. Is it a disturbance of the release of iron from the macrophage system to the circulation or is it true iron deficiency? I think you have to start doing bone marrow biopsies and stain them to have a better idea of the actual iron status of these patients.

Kühn: Coming back to the question of Dr. Müller-Wiefel: Within the group of reduced responders, where we assumed iron deficiency, 2 patients were included who responded to i.v. iron substitution alone without an additional increase in EPO dose. We only had to give them i.v. iron supplementation without raising the EPO dose.

Hampl (Berlin): I want to pose a question to the auditorium. Is it clever to interrupt desferrioxamine therapy of patients with aluminum intoxication during treatment with EPO? I think not. What do you think? You and the auditorium?

Kühn: I really have no experience. But a couple of weeks ago, there appeared a paper from Casati. He reported that he found an inverse relation between hematocrit response and aluminum plasma levels after desferrioxamine challenge. He decided not to stop EPO therapy in aluminum-loaded patients, but increased the EPO dose and finally had success. So, I would conclude from his experience that it is not necessary to stop EPO therapy in patients who are aluminum overloaded.

Winearls (London): You said your patients are not aluminum toxic. Can I ask first what you define as aluminum toxicity?

Kühn: The only parameter studied in our patients were aluminum plasma levels. We did not perform bone marrow staining and the desferrioxamine test as Casati has done.

Winearls: I have a problem with Casati's data. He claimed that there was a relationship between the peak dose of EPO that the patients reached and the delta-aluminum after desferrioxamine challenge. What we do not know from Casati's data is whether the maintenance dose of EPO required by those patients was related to their delta-aluminum. In discussing reasons for failure to respond we should try to define aluminum toxicity so that it can be treated before concluding that the EPO dose is inadequate.

Klinkmann: Thank you very much for this suggestions. We tried in West Berlin during the EDTA meeting to arrive at some approximate definition of aluminum toxicity. It is obviously almost impossible but I think we should come back to our question because, before continuing, it would be useful to have some sort of definition.

Waters: Could you imagine that the nonresponsiveness could be due to a transient depletion of transferrin itself by infection.

Kühn: I should hand over this question to Dr. Bommer. You had a patient with nonresponse and infection.

Bommer: It was a patient who had urinary tract infection. I cannot give you the exact data of the transferrin during this period. I must look for it. I cannot remember a significant fall of transferrin.

Hampl: We had 1 patient with reduced response and this was a patient with aluminum intoxication as proven by bone biopsy after tetracycline staining. We interrupted the desferrioxamine therapy at the beginning of EPO treatment and I think this was wrong. When the next case comes up I think it will be better to continue with desferrioxamine during the EPO therapy.

Auditorium: Why?

Hampl: Because I think it is not good that we have aluminum in a patient and because of this have to give more EPO. Perhaps, if we give desferrioxamine at the same time the response to EPO would be better.

Klinkmann: It is difficult for the chairman to differentiate between hypothesis and speculation.

Hampl: Yes!

Eschbach: I would like to plead that we study these patients very carefully. My understanding is that your protocol excluded anybody with a mean corpuscular volume below 80. Is that right?

Kühn: Yes.

Eschbach: No one has treated and studied many aluminum toxic patients who had microcytosis, so we do not know whether they will respond to rhEPO. The issue is, does aluminum overload, whether associated with normocytic or microcytic red cells, interfer with rhEPO responsiveness? We also need to know what is the best way to define aluminum overload: DFO challenge, bone-biopsy, or both. To muddy the water with concomitant use of rhEPO and DFO in patients with questionable aluminum overload is not going to answer the question.

Klinkmann: I fully agree and I conclude from this meeting for all future studies that this issue should be very carefully looked at and investigated.

Contr. Nephrol., vol. 66, pp. 104–113 (Karger, Basel 1988)

Beneficial and Adverse Effects of Correction of Anaemia by Recombinant Human Erythropoietin in Patients on Maintenance Haemodialysis

P. Grützmacher[a], *M. Bergmann*[a], *T. Weinreich*[b], *U. Nattermann*[c], *E. Reimers*[d], *M. Pollok*[e]

Departments of Nephrology, University Hospitals of [a]Frankfurt/M., [b]Heidelberg, [c]Munich, [d]Hannover and [e]Cologne, FRG

The development of recombinant human erythropoietin (rhEPO) offered for the first time a possibility of an effective and continous correction of the anaemia of patients with end-stage renal disease. However, in two pioneer trials [Winearls et al., 1986; Eschbach et al., 1987], correction of anaemia was accompanied by several adverse effects and occasionally severe complications; a causative relationship to rhEPO therapy was assumed in some cases. Apart from minor subjective discomfort, an increase of the serum levels of urea, creatinine and potassium as well as an increase of blood pressure was observed in some patients. Unexpected hyperkalaemia and worsening of hypertension was life-threatening in some cases. It seems suggestive that most of the adverse effects of this new treatment were not related to substance-specific effects of rhEPO itself, but secondary to the correction of anaemia. The beneficial and adverse effects of a German multicentre study are reported in the following.

Patients and Parameters Investigated

The clinical and side effects, observed in the rhEPO multicentre study, are reported with the exception of the effects on blood pressure, which are described separately in the paper by Samtleben [1988]. The design of the trial has been described before in this issue [Bommer, 1988]. Regular haemodialysis patients were treated in a randomized fashion with either 40, 80, or 120 U rhEPO intravenously thrice weekly. Evaluation of the initial treatment period (correction period) was based upon the data of 92 patients, 85 of these

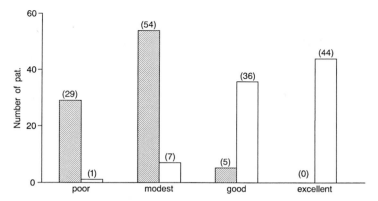

Fig. 1. Effect of rhEPO therapy on physical fitness in patients on maintenance haemodialysis. ▨ = Run-in period; ▢ = rhEPO therapy (end of dose-finding period).

being treated for more than 12 weeks. The patients were regularly interviewed about potential subjective complaints and their well-being by the attending physicians. Serum chemistry, including electrolytes, urea, creatinine, bilirubin, liver enzymes, and lactate dehydrogenase (LHD) were controlled weekly at the end of the long interdialytic period. Total protein, albumin, electrophoresis, acid-base status, and blood coagulation parameters were controlled monthly. Serum ferritin concentration was determined every fortnight. Thrombocytes and whole as well as differential white blood cell counts were controlled weekly. Changes in medical and haemodialysis therapy, including body weight, dialysis time, potassium concentration in the dialysis fluid and heparinization were recorded regularly.

Results

The physical fitness of 88 of the 92 patients was classified into four categories by the attending physicians prior to rhEPO therapy: before rhEPO, 29 patients were in a poor condition (frequently disabled, needing assistance); 54 patients were in a moderate condition (able to walk and to care for themselves); only 5 patients were in a good condition (enabling professional work), and no patient was in an excellent condition (feeling no real limitation of physical activity during efforts of usual everyday life).

Under rhEPO therapy, a considerable improvement of physical condition and well-being was observed in most of the patients (fig. 1). An increase of appetite was reported frequently. However, the mean body weight of the three groups did not change. The importance of the improved physical fitness for the patients' life is illustrated by the following four examples:

Table I. Serum chemistry during rhEPO therapy in patients on maintenance haemodialysis, median and range (in parentheses)

	Run-in (mean of all values) n = 92	Last value correction period or week 12 n = 92	Last value maintenance period, 18–28 weeks after start of rhEPO n = 62
Sodium, mmol/l	139 (127–150)	140 (120–156)	138 (123–147)
Potassium, mmol/l	5.5 (3.7–8.0)	5.6 (3.7–7.8)	5.7 (3.8–7.7)
Calcium, mmol/l	2.4 (1.8–2.8)	2.4 (2.0–3.0)	2.4 (2.0–4.8)
Phosphate, mmol/l	1.8 (0.4–3.3)	2.0 (0.4–3.3)	1.9 (0.6–3.0)
Alkaline phosphatase, U/l	111 (44–361)	119 (43–472)	123 (46–655)
SGPT, U/l	8 (3–74)	8 (1–86)	8 (4–83)
SGOT, U/l	7 (2–32)	7 (2–26)	7 (3–86)
Gamma-GT	10 (2–91)	10 (2–107)	8 (1–84)

Case 1: A 52-year-old patient, mother of several children in a previously disabled physical condition, needing home care – now fully rehabilitated, able to care for her family.

Case 2: A 51-year-old patient in a poor physical condition, due to severe coronary heart disease with angina of effort – now working as a bricklayer in his leisure time.

Case 3: A 67-year-old veteran sportsman in a bad condition – meanwhile the patient has taken up bicycle riding.

Case 4: A 27-year-old female patient in a poor physical condition, always complaining of tiredness and fatigue – meanwhile the patient has recommenced professional work as a bookbinder, and plays squash.

A marked improvement of wound healing was observed in 2 patients with previously persisting defects.

Blood and serum chemistry is shown in tables I and II. The median serum levels of potassium and phosphate remained unchanged in all groups. In a few cases an increase of potassium level during rhEPO therapy was observed. The median serum concentrations of urea and creatinine of the three groups did not change either. Furthermore, no change was found for bilirubin, liver enzymes and LDH. However, dialysis time was increased in 10 patients due to deterioration of either electrolytes or retention products. The potassium concentration of the dialysis fluid was lowered occasionally. In 1 patient with potassium levels of 6.5–7.0 mmol/l prior to rhEPO, hyperkalaemia of 8.5 mmol/l necessitated an additional dialysis after sev-

Table II. Serum and blood chemistry under rhEPO therapy in patients on maintenance haemodialysis, median and range (in parentheses)

	Run-in (mean of all values) n = 92	Last value correction period or week 12 n = 92	Last value maintenance period, 18–28 weeks after start of rhEPO n = 62
LDH, U/l	142 (27–214)	138 (85–334)	145 (62–260)
Total protein, g/dl	6.8 (5.3–8.6)	6.8 (5.5–9.9)	6.8 (5.9–8.4)
Creatinine, mg/dl	12.1 (5.6–18.7)	11.8 (5.5–17.8)	12.4 (5.9–19.1)
Urea, mg/dl	163 (88–270)	165 (58–302)	176 (46–261)
pH	7.34 (7.15–7.43)	7.31 (7.13–7.46)	7.31 (6.96–7.44)
Prothrombin time, %	92 (32–100)	98 (29–100)	90 (27–116)
Partial thromboplastin time, sec	33 (20–64)	31 (20–90)	32 (22–101)

eral weeks of treatment. The mean daily dose of oral phosphate binders remained constant.

In figures 2 and 3 pretreatment values of serum ferritin concentrations and thrombocyte counts are compared with those observed during the first 4 treatment weeks and at the end of the correction period or week 12 before patients were put on rhEPO maintenance doses. Along with the increase of haematocrit, a considerable decrease of serum iron and ferritin levels was observed (fig. 2), necessitating iron supplementation in nearly all patients. Relative iron deficiency characterized by an almost complete standstill of the previously increasing haematocrit in the presence of serum ferritin levels in the lower normal range occurred frequently. Currently, the majority of the patients require iron supplementation.

During rhEPO treatment, in the majority of the patients a moderate increase of thrombocyte counts could be observed. In comparison with the median pretreatment values the corresponding values at the end of the correction period were significantly higher in all treatment groups ($p < 0.05$, distribution-free signed Wilcoxon rank test) (fig. 3). True thrombocytosis was observed in 4 patients; 1 of these presented with thrombocytosis prior to rhEPO therapy. In the remaining 3 patients the effect was transitory and not associated with any complications. Whole and differential white blood cell counts remained unaffected.

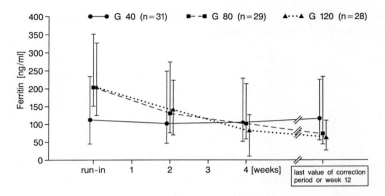

Fig. 2. Serum ferritin levels during rhEPO therapy in patients on maintenance haemodialysis (median and interquartile range). The increase of serum ferritin levels at the end of the dose-finding period is due to an enhanced iron supplementation in the majority of the patients in order to promote correction of anaemia. G 40, G 80, and G 120 indicate the 3 treatment groups receiving thrice weekly doses of 40, 80, and 120 U of rhEPO, respectively.

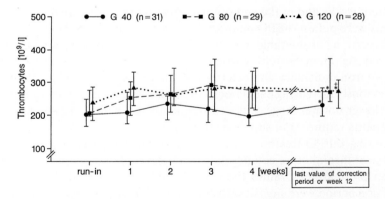

Fig. 3. Effect of rhEPO therapy on thrombocyte counts in patients on maintenance haemodialysis (medium and interquartile range). G 40, G 80, and G 120 indicate the 3 treatment groups receiving thrice weekly doses of 40, 80, and 120 U of rhEPO, respectively. * = Significantly different from pretreatment value (average of run-in), $p < 0.05$, distribution-free signed Wilcoxon rank test. + = Significantly different from G 40 at week 12, $p < 0.05$, distribution-free signed Wilcoxon rank sum test.

Thrombosis of the arteriovenous fistula occurred in 5 of 92 patients, 4 of these being fistulae on risk with more than one previous occlusion. No other thromboembolic events have been observed. Occlusion of the dialyzer system was rarely reported and did not seem to be more frequent than before initiation of rhEPO therapy. It has to be considered however that in 35 of 92 patients the dosage of heparin used for haemodialysis was increased, resulting in an increase of the median heparin dose by about 1,000 units per session in every treatment group.

Currently surveying more than 7,500 injections and a treatment time of 26–34 weeks, therapy with rhEPO was tolerated well. There were no problems of local intolerance. Intracutaneous testings, performed in each case with a dose of 20 units before the first intravenous application, were all negative, except in 1 patient, where a slight early reaction was observed. A repetition of the test showed the same result in this case. In spite of this, the patient tolerated intravenous therapy well.

Due to systemic intolerance, rhEPO therapy was interrupted in 2 patients: the first patient complained about weakness and pain in the joints already after the first injection. After the third injection, therapy had to be discontinued. The second patient complained of recurrent headache in the presence of a normal blood pressure always after EPO injection; symptoms developed after more than 8 weeks of rhEPO therapy. Another patient complained about nausea after EPO infusion; after prolongation of infusion time, symptoms disappeared completely.

Transitory influenza-like symptoms occurred in 5 patients. Occasionally, sweating, paraesthesias in the legs and a feeling of warmth was reported. Exacerbation of common acne was observed in 4 patients, returning to the initial status under long-term therapy.

During the treatment phase, the following major clinical events occurred: A 61-year-old male presented with headache and spastic hemiplegia due to a subdural haematoma, which was removed surgically resulting in a complete restitution. This complication occurred 11 days after the beginning of treatment in the presence of a normal blood pressure and a minor increase in haematocrit. Coagulation parameters were normal. A patient with severe coronary heart disease and status after myocardial infarction and fourfold aortocoronary bypass operation prior to rhEPO therapy needed resuscitation after a collapse of unclear origin after 16 weeks of treatment, with an increase of haematocrit from 18 to 30%. He recovered completely. This patient had suffered from severe ventricular arrhythmias prior to therapy. One 70-year-old diabetic male with a chronically increased intraocular pressure suffered from acute glaucoma after correction of anaemia. In 1 patient, a non-A-, non-B-hepatitis developed after less than 8 weeks of rhEPO therapy. A causative relationship seems unlikely in all the above examples. All major clinical events related to increases of blood pressure are reported separately [Samtleben, 1988].

Discussion

The present results show that correction of renal anaemia in RDT patients results in a marked improvement in patients' physical fitness and well-being. This effect has been confirmed in other studies [Winearls et al., 1986; Eschbach et al., 1987; Bommer et al., 1987]. As the examples demonstrate, the continuous correction of renal anaemia impressively altered patients' life under medical and social aspects. The improvement of well-being suggests that renal anaemia is rather tolerated than compensated in most of these patients.

The effective increase of red blood cell generation is associated with a considerably increased demand of iron, as shown by the evident decrease of serum ferritin levels. The development of functional or absolute iron deficiency may hamper an effective correction of renal anaemia [Eschbach et al., 1987], requiring a close monitoring of serum iron and ferritin levels under rhEPO therapy. In the present trial, iron supplementation had to be increased in most of the patients.

The question whether the stimulatory effect of rhEPO is restricted to the red cell line is of considerable clinical importance. There is evidence from in vitro studies that rhEPO exerts some stimulatory effects on murine megakaryocytes [Ishibashi et al., 1987]; other studies using human progenitor cells did not confirm this observation [Ganser et al., 1987]. In the first two clinical trials [Winearls et al., 1986; Eschbach et al., 1987] no effect on thrombocyte counts was observed; however, in a following study an increase of the median thrombocyte count during rhEPO therapy was reported [Bommer et al., 1987]. The results of the present study clearly demonstrate a stimulatory effect of rhEPO on thrombocyte counts in RDT patients. It is of special importance that this effect was dose related and developed only with dosages used for the correction of anaemia. The data evaluated so far indicate that this effect disappears with lower rhEPO doses during the maintenance phase. True thrombocytosis developed rarely and was not associated with complications. Thrombosis of the arteriovenous fistula, observed in 5 of the patients, did not appear to be more frequent than usual, considering that 4 of these where high risk fistulas with antecedent thrombotic occlusions due to stenoses, while no other thromboembolic events have been observed up to now. Occlusions of the dialyzer system were rarely reported. However, in 40% of the patients, the amount of heparin required for dialysis was increased moderately.

The increase of serum levels of retention products and potassium observed in other studies [Winearls et al., 1986; Eschbach et al., 1987] could not be confirmed. Statistical analysis of the median changes of potassium, phosphate, urea and creatinine of the three different groups showed no significant changes. However, it has to be considered that dialysis time was prolonged in 10 of the 92 patients. Furthermore, patients were regularly advised to adhere to a low potassium diet and underwent closer controls as usual. In some individual cases, an increase of potassium, partially accompanied by a less pronounced increase of urea and creatinine, was noted. The increase of potassium and other retention products may be attributed to dietary changes, as the patients frequently reported an increased appetite. There was no evidence for an increased haemolysis, as reflected by unchanged LDH levels. A simultaneous increase of serum creatinine levels suggests a reduced dialysis efficacy, as an increase in haemotocrit necessarily leads to a decreased dialyzer plasma flow if blood flow remains constant [Babb et al., 1972]. However, dialysis efficacy was not measured in this study.

Although therapy with rhEPO is well tolerated in general, an intracutaneous test before the first intravenous application is still recommended. As the data show, a negative intracutaneous result does not exclude intravenous intolerance, which has been observed in 2 patients in this study. Influenza-like symptoms observed in some patients were always transitory, so that all of these patients decided to continue rhEPO treatment. The mechanisms of the exacerbation of common acne are still unclear. Androgen metabolism may be influenced by rhEPO, because rhEPO probably exerts certain anabolic effects, as reflected by the increased appetite. Experience of long-term therapy will enable a definite judgement.

References

Babb, A. L.; Popovich, R. P.; Farrell, T. C.; Blagg, C. R.: The effects of erythrocyte mass transfer rates on solute clearance measurements during haemodialysis. Proc. Eur. Dial. Transplant Ass. 9: 505–521 (1972).

Bommer, J.; Müller-Bühl, E.; Ritz, E.; Eifert, J.: Recombinant human erythropoietin in anaemic patients on haemodialysis (letter). Lancet i: 392 (1987).

Bommer, J.; Kugel, M.; Schoeppe, W.; Brunkhorst, R.; Samtleben, W.; Bramsiepe, P.; Scigalla, P.: Dose-related effects of recombinant human erythropoietin on erythropoiesis. Contr. Nephrol., vol. 66, pp. 85–93 (Karger, Basel 1988).

Eschbach, J. W.; Egrie, J. C.; Downing, M. R.; Browne, J. K.; Adamson, J. W.: Correction of the anemia of end-stage renal disease with recombinant human erythropoietin. New Engl. J. Med. *316:* 73–78 (1987).

Ganser, A., Voelkers, B.; Scigalla, P.; Hoelzer, D.: Effects of recombinant human erythropoietin on human hematopoietic progenitor cells (abstract). Proc. Xth Int. Congr. Nephrol., London 1987.

Ishibashi, T.; Koziol, J. A.; Burstein, S. A.: Human recombinant erythropoietin promotes differentiation of murine megakaryocytes in vitro. J. clin. Invest. *79:* 286–289 (1987).

Samtleben, W., Baldamus, C. A.; Bommer, J.; Fassbinder, W.; Nonnast-Daniel, B.; Gurland, H. J.: Blood pressure changes during treatment with recombinant human erythropoietin. Contr. Nephrol., vol. 66, pp. 114–122 (Karger, Basel 1988).

Winearls, C. G.; Oliver, D. O.; Pippard, M. J.; Reid, C.; Downing, M. R.; Cotes, P. M.: Effect of human erythropoietin derived from recombinant DNA on the anaemia of patients maintained by chronic haemodialysis. Lancet *ii:* 1175–1178 (1986).

Peter Grützmacher, MD, Department of Nephrology, Division of Internal Medicine, University Hospital, Theodor-Stern-Kai 7, D–6000 Frankfurt/M. (FRG)

Discussion

Ehrich (Hannover): Was iron deficiency intercorrelated with thrombocytosis? Because it is known that you may have thrombocytosis in iron deficiency?

Grützmacher: We did not have this impression. I think we should look again at our data under this aspect.

Stummvoll (Linz): We had some rise in blood pressure immediately after the injection of erythropoietin. Did you see this? Not hematocrit dependent, but immediately after the injection of EPO.

Grützmacher: I think we should delegate the answer to this question to Dr. Samtleben after his talk.

Bergström (Huddinge): Could you elaborate on the reason why the patients get hyperkalemic and hyperphosphatemic? Has this something to do with the increased intake of protein or something else?

Grützmacher: It is a matter of speculation. From a statistical point of view we cannot support these observations because there was no significant change of the median values. This does not exclude relevant changes in individual patients. Let us focus on the deterioration of these products. An increase of potassium as well as phosphate might, on a theoretical basis, be caused by an absolute increase of hemolysis due to an increased number of erythrocytes with an unchanged and still shortened red cell survival time. However, we have no clinical evidence for an increased hemolysis in this study. Regarding urea, it might well be, as reflected by the increase of appetite, that these patients have a higher intake of protein. But on a multicenter basis, we have measured neither protein catabolic rate nor dietary changes. We have the impression – as in the case I showed you –

that the increase of potassium was mostly associated with an increase of creatinine and urea. This suggests worsening of dialysis efficacy. If you keep the blood flow constant and increase the hematocrit, the plasma flow must go down. However, we have not performed any measurements.

Bergström: I feel it is very important that we learn more about this. The impression from our first patient is that the intake of protein has increased very much during EPO treatment. We have also seen an improvement in the protein DNA ratio in muscle tissue which is a good indication that the patient is anabolic.

Grützmacher: This should lead to an increase in dry body weight; however, in this study there was no increase in mean body weight after dialysis.

Bauer (Zürich): An effect of EPO on the thrombocyte count would suggest that erythropoietin is also thrombopoietin. Would you like to comment on this?

Grützmacher: The study of Ishibashi, which is an in vitro cell culture study, shows that erythropoietin stimulates thrombocyte metabolism and that erythropoietin added to cell cultures results in an enlargement of megakaryocytes. I think Dr. Ganser in the last talk will have further information about the effect of erythroipoietin on stem cells and megakaryocytes.

Bauer: Would you expect an effect on megakaryocytes?

Grützmacher: Probably EPO has an effect on the development of this cell line. But I think we should wait for Dr. Ganser's results.

Klinkmann (Rostock): Coming from the institution of Viktor Schilling, the father of the white blood count, I would like to remind you that Schilling already in 1936 or 1937 pointed out that with any kind of improved erythropoiesis there is also an improvement of thrombopoiesis. At that time it was a clear clinical observation for which we now may find new evidence.

Eschbach: Two comments: (1) Not everybody has shown an increase in the platelet count as you have. The increase that has occurred, although statistically significant, is still within the normal range. It appears that long-term treatment does not cause any further increase in platelet counts. I am not sure whether this has any clinical relevance, although it is conceivable that it may relate to the increased heparin requirements the patients require. (2) The second point has to do with the rise in serum potassium. I originally thought this was from increased food intake. Our dieticians have tried to document this but it is difficult to get a good dietary history. There is no increase in hemolysis. On the other hand, the red cell mass is doubled in some instances, so there is an increased potassium load generated when these cells die. But I don't know whether that is a significant potassium load. I welcome the thoughts of others.

Kurtz: You mentioned that you had to interrupt therapy in 1 patient because of development of headache. Is this a real side effect or what is the incidence of spontaneous development of headache in patients? Because in single cases it is really the question whether it is a side effect or a spontaneous, independent development.

Grützmacher: In this case, headaches occurred always after the injection of erythropoietin. But this was seen after more than 8 weeks' of treatment. The first 8 weeks were uneventful.

Contr. Nephrol., vol. 66, pp. 114–122 (Karger, Basel 1988)

Blood Pressure Changes during Treatment with Recombinant Human Erythropoietin

W. Samtleben[a], *C. A. Baldamus*[b], *J. Bommer*[c], *W. Fassbinder*[d], *B. Nonnast-Daniel*[e], *H. J. Gurland*[a]

[a]Nephrology Division, Medical Clinic I, Klinikum München-Grosshadern, Ludwigs-Maximilians University, München; [b]Medical Clinic, University of Cologne, Cologne; [c]Medical Clinic, University of Heidelberg, Heidelberg; [d]Department of Internal Medicine, Johann Wolfgang Goethe University Frankfurt, Frankfurt/Main, and [e]Nephrology Division, Department of Internal Medicine, Medizinische Hochschule Hannover, Hannover, FRG

The correction of renal anemia with recombinant human erythropoietin (rhEPO) opens a new dimension in the treatment of end-stage renal disease by dialysis. As with other effective therapeutic regimens, treatment with rhEPO is associated with side effects which have to be managed or which may limit its application. Side effects reported so far include a worsening of hypertension [1–4], hypertensive encephalopathy sometimes with seizures [1, 2, 4], fistula clotting [1, 4, 5], hyperkalemia [2, 4], and a rise in serum urea [2]. In the sparse literature on the therapeutic application of rhEPO [1–7], hypertension has been described to worsen or to become evident in 0–70% of the patients treated (table I) [1–5]. Two studies with 13 and 67 patients respectively found no side effects; however, they did not specifically refer to blood pressure [6, 7]. Here, we analyze the blood pressure changes observed in the dialysis patients treated in a multicenter study in the FRG. The study design has been described in detail elsewhere [8]. Based on the known side effects, uncontrolled hypertension, but not a manageable rise in blood pressure, was an exclusion criterion for entry into this multicenter study.

Patients

Ninety-five patients regularly treated with intermittent hemodialysis entered the multicenter study. Data from 3 patients were incomplete and could not be included in the

Table I. Effect of rhEPO on blood pressure (literature overview)

Reference	Patients treated with an effective dose, n	Patients with blood pressure increase, n	rhEPO dose range U/kg b.w.
Bommer et al., 1987 [3]	13	9	24–192
Casati et al., 1987 [4]	14	8	24–192
Eschbach et al., 1987 [2]	18	4	15–500
Stutz et al., 1987 [5]	8	0	24–192
Urabe et al., 1987 [6]	67	?	6–200
Winearls et al., 1986 [1]	10	1	3–192
Zins et al., 1986 [5]	13	?	24–192

Table II. Primary renal diseases of all patients including the hypertensive group enrolled in the multicenter rhEPO study

	Patients, n	Hypertensive patients, n
Glomerular disease	36	21
Pyelonephritis	21	6
Hereditary nephropathy	5	4
Diabetic nephropathy	6	3
Other	24	11

evaluation. Of the remaining 92 dialysis patients, 2 were hypotensive, 45 were normotensive without any medication, while 45 were hypertensive or required antihypertensive medication. The distribution of primary renal diseases in the hypertensive group was not different from the study population as a whole (table II). The following analysis is based on an evaluation of the predialysis blood pressure, including the systolic, diastolic and mean arterial blood pressures.

Results

The systolic, diastolic and mean arterial blood pressures (mean value and range) at the start of the study were not different between the three subgroups, later treated with 40, 80 or 120 U rhEPO/kg b.w. according to the randomization protocol (table III). The data in table IV show the changes in blood pressure during the initial period of the study when hematocrits were

Table III. Blood pressure at start of study with respect to rhEPO dose; median (range)

	Randomization groups		
	40 U/rhEPO/kg	80 U/rhEPO/kg	120 U/rhEPO/kg
Systolic blood pressure, mm Hg	141 (87–180)	140 (100–178)	139 (109–164)
Diastolic blood pressure, mm Hg	77 (43–101)	78 (57–96)	77 (67–91)
Mean arterial pressure, mm Hg	123 (72–156)	125 (90–154)	124 (106–140)

Table IV. Blood pressure changes in patients on rhEPO therapy at the end of the correction phase; median (range)

	Systolic blood pressure, mm Hg	Diastolic blood pressure, mm Hg	Mean arterial blood pressure, mm Hg
40 U/kg b.w.	+1.5 (–25 to +46.5)	+5.4 (–40.9 to +40.0)	+5.3 (–33.9 to +29.8
80 U/kg b.w.	–1.8 (–13.6 to +20.4)	+1.3 (–19.2 to +20.5)	+0.8 (–17.0 to +16.8)
120 U/kg b.w.	+4.5 (–29.6 to +37.5)	+5.3 (–28.6 to +34.6)	+5.9 (–24.7 to +30.7)

increased from a median prestudy level of 22% (range 16–28%) to their steady-state level of 30–35%. Overall, the blood pressure changes observed in the three groups during this phase were comparable for all three evaluated parameters (systolic, diastolic, and mean arterial blood pressure). However, this analysis compares the treatment groups as a whole and does not take into account individual blood pressure changes or any therapeutic interventions required because of an increasing blood pressure.

At least 3 of 92 patients experienced interdialytic hypertensive episodes. This figure may underestimate the actual incidence of interdialytic hypertension, as no regular blood pressure readings were obtained interdialytically.

Examination of the therapeutic interventions in response to blood pressure changes shows that in 6 of the 45 originally normotensive patients antihypertensive drug treatment had to be initiated. Furthermore, 21 out of the 45 initially hypertensive patients required a more intensive antihyper-

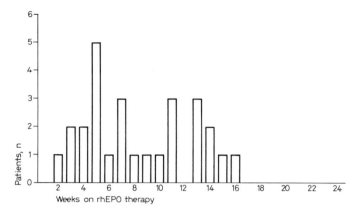

Fig. 1. Weeks on rhEPO therapy when antihypertensive medication was started or increased.

tensive regimen to control their blood pressure. In contrast, 2 patients, originally hypertensive, were able to have their medications withdrawn.

An increase in blood pressure requiring an intensification of antihypertensive therapy was first seen 2 weeks after the first rhEPO infusion (fig. 1). After 16 weeks of rhEPO therapy, blood pressure was controlled in all study patients and no further vigorous changes in antihypertensive medication were required. The drugs preferentially used for treatment of hypertension included nifedipine, vasodilators, betablockers, and angiotensin-converting enzyme blockers.

No correlation could be found between the increasing blood pressure and the rhEPO dose administered, or the weekly increase in hematocrit, or the absolute platelet count.

Due to the problems with the management of hypertension, rhEPO therapy was stopped in 3 patients. Furthermore, 1 patient died during the study period, probably as a consequence of a severe hypertensive episode.

Case Reports

Case 1. Patient A. O. (born 1926) had been on hemodialysis for more than 3 years before rhEPO therapy was started. His primary renal disease was chronic glomerulonephritis. When dialysis was initiated he was hypertensive and severely anemic. In 1984,

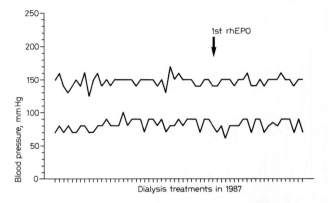

Fig. 2. Time course of blood pressure (predialysis, systolic and diastolic) in patient A. O.

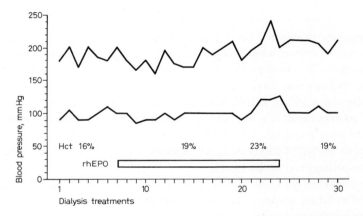

Fig. 3. Time course of blood pressure (predialysis, systolic and diastolic) and hematocrit in patient A. W.

coronary angiography was performed which showed mild coronary atherosclerotic lesions. In May 1985, a stenosis of both carotid arteries was diagnosed and a bypass operation performed on the right side. In June 1986, he had a cardiopulmonary arrest at home. He was successfully resuscitated and a few hours later his blood pressure had stabilized at 220/120 mm Hg. Following this, he recovered completely and his blood pressure was kept normal with mild antihypertensive therapy. As his hematocrit was persistently low he was included in the rhEPO study (first rhEPO infusion in April 1987). During all study phases (rhEPO dosage 120 U/kg b.w.), his blood pressure did not show any significant change (fig. 2), however, 6 weeks after rhEPO was first administered, a second cardiopulmonary

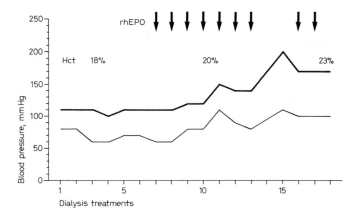

Fig. 4. Time course of blood pressure (predialysis, systolic and diastolic) and hematocrit in patient I. C.

arrest occurred. After successful resuscitation he was admitted to a community hospital. At that time, his systolic blood pressure was 200–250 mmHg, requiring continuous intravenous infusion of antihypertensives. Despite intensive therapy his cerebral status did not recover and renal replacement therapy was terminated. No autopsy was performed.

Case 2. Patient A. W. (born 1961) has been on renal replacement therapy since October 1986. His underlying renal disease is minimal change glomerulopathy with relapsing episodes of nephrotic syndrome since 1964. After being stable for more than 6 months on intermittent hemodialysis, he was enrolled in the rhEPO study. At that time, his predialysis blood pressure was controlled by antihypertensive medication (betablockers and nifedipine). Before entering the rhEPO study, progressive increases in his blood pressure were observed in several dialysis sessions. These responded promptly to the administration of 10–20 mg nifedipine orally. Because of a slowly increasing predialysis blood pressure (fig. 3), his dialysis treatment time was prolonged from 4 to 5 h per session. After 6 weeks of rhEPO (40 U/kg b.w.) therapy, hypertensive episodes with systolic pressures of 210–240 mm Hg 10–20 min postdialysis were observed. This prompted us to stop the hormone replacement therapy. Although the pre- and postdialysis blood pressure profile did not change in the following weeks, no further hypertensive episodes of the same severity were observed.

Case 3. Patient I. C. (born 1956) developed end-stage renal failure due to membranous glomerulonephritis. Dialysis was started in 1985. His blood pressure was normalized with a combination of dialysis (3×5 h) and prazosin. After 2 weeks on rhEPO therapy (120 U/kg b.w.), his predialysis blood pressure began to increase with peak values of 200 mm Hg systolic (fig. 4) requiring additional medication. At that time his hematocrit had increased by only 5 vol%. Because of preexisting cardiomyopathy, it was decided to stop rhEPO therapy and within 3 weeks his blood pressure had returned to normal.

Comment

Case 1 was a high risk patient with preexisting coronary heart disease and carotid artery stenoses as well as a previous history of a cardiovascular arrest. In this case, a relationship between rhEPO therapy and death is most uncertain. In case 2, a relationship between the hypertensive episodes and rhEPO is also questionable. However, in case 3 and in a fourth patient withdrawn from the study, a causal relationship between rhEPO and hypertension is likely.

Discussion

Our data do not support a direct hypertensive effect of rhEPO; however, hypertension worsened in 21 out of 45 hypertensive patients (47%) and developed in 6 out of 45 previously normotensive patients (13%). The incidence of hypertensive complications obviously depends on patient selection and this can explain the widely variable incidence (0–70%) of an increasing blood pressure described in patients treated with rhEPO [1–5]. Except for preexisting hypertension, we could identify no other risk factors for the development or worsening of hypertension. In all but 3 cases, hypertension could be managed with additional medication, using beta-blockers, nifedipine, angiotensin-converting enzyme blockers or clonidine. Hypertension was a problem only during the initial 4 months of rhEPO therapy. Thereafter, blood pressures remained stable and did not require further therapeutic interventions (observation period so far 7 months). The one death observed in our study cannot be attributed with any certainty to the rhEPO therapy. The incidence of one death in 92 severely anemic dialysis patients is below the overall mortality rate described for dialysis patients [9, 10], most likely because of the very strict criteria applied for entry into this study.

References

1 Winearls, C. G.; Oliver, D. O.; Pippard, M. J.; Reid, C.; Downing, M. R.; Cotes, P. M.: Effect of human erythropoietin derived from recombinant DNA on the anaemia of patients maintained by chronic haemodialysis. Lancet *ii:* 1175–1178 (1986).
2 Eschbach, J. W.; Egrie, J. C.; Downing, M. R.; Browne, J. K.; Adamson, J. W.: Correction of the anemia of end-stage renal disease with recombinant human ery-

thropoietin. Results of a combined phase I and II clinical trial. New Engl. J. Med. *316:* 73–78 (1987).

3   Bommer, J.; Alexiou, C.; Müller-Bühl, U.; Eifert, J.: Ritz, E.: Recombinant human erythropoietin therapy in haemodialysis patients – dose determination and clinical experience. Nephrol. Dial. Transplant. *2:* 238–242 (1987).

4   Casati, S.; Passerini, P.; Campise, M. R.; Graziani, G.; Cesana, B.; Peresic, M.; Ponticelli, C.: Benefits and risks of protracted treatment with human recombinant erythropoietin in patients having haemodialysis. Br. med. J. *295:* 1017–1020 (1987).

5   Stutz, B.; Rhyner, K.; Vögtli, J.; Binswanger, U.: Erfolgreiche Behandlung der Anämie bei Hämodialyse-Patienten mit rekombiniertem humanem Erythropoietin. Erhaltungsdosis und Serumkonzentration. Schweiz. med. Wschr. *117:* 1397–1402 (1987).

6   Zins, B.; Drüeke, T.; Zingraff, J.; Bererhi, L.; Kreis, H.; Naret, C.; Delons, S.; Castaigne, J.-P.; Peterlongo, F.; Casadevall, N.; Varet, B.: Erythropoietin treatment in anaemic patients on haemodialysis (Letter to the editor). Lancet *ii:* 1329 (1986).

7   Urabe, A.; Takaku, F.; Mimura, N.: Therapeutic effect of recombinant human erythropoietin on anemia caused by chronic renal disease (Abstract). Exp. Hematol. *15:* 438 (1987).

8   Bommer, J.; Kugel, M.; Schoeppe, W.; Brunkhorst, R.; Samtleben, W.; Bramsiepe, P.; Scigalla, P.: Dose-related effects of recombinant human erythropoietin on erythropoiesis. Contr. Nephrol., vol. 66, pp. 85–93 (Karger, Basel 1988).

9   Brynger, H.; Brunner, F. P.; Chantler, C.; Donckerwolcke, R. A.; Jacobs, C.; Kramer, P.; Selwood, N. H.; Wing, A. J.: Combined report on regular dialysis and transplantation in Europe, X, 1979. Proc. Eur. Dial. Transplant Ass. *17:* 2–84 (1980).

10 Wing, A. J.; Broyer, M.; Brunner, F. P.; Brynger, H.; Challah, S.; Donckerwolcke, R. A.; Gretz, N.; Jacobs, C.; Kramer, P.; Selwood, N. H.: Combined report on regular dialysis and transplantation in Europe, XIII, 1982. Proc. Eur. Dial. Transplant Ass. *20:* 2–71 (1983).

Priv. Doz. Dr. med. Walter Samtleben, Nephrology Division, Medical Clinic I, University Hospital München-Grosshadern, POB 701 260, D-8000 München 70 (FRG)

Discussion

Wizemann (Giessen): Did the incidence of symptomatic hypotension during dialysis change when the patients had reached the goal hematocrit between 30 and 35%?

Samtleben: The blood pressure behavior during the dialysis sessions, and especially the hypotensive episodes, were not a parameter for evaluation in this study. Therefore, I can only refer to the patients from our center and there I do not have the impression of a different blood pressure profile during the dialysis treatment before and after correction of anemia. In general, hypotensive episodes are rare in our center.

Klinkmann (Rostock): What Dr. Wizemann is really asking for is the incidence of hypotensive episodes during dialysis.

Samtleben: As I said, hypotensive episodes are rare in our center.

Stummvoll (Linz): Do you have any statistical data of blood pressure pre- and post-erythropoietin (EPO) administration?

Samtleben: Evaluation criteria were blood pressures at the beginning and at the end of each dialysis session. After termination of the dialysis treatment, patients received the EPO infusion. We did not routinely measure the blood pressure at the end of the EPO infusion, but in those patients who developed headache or other symptoms we did. One of our patients exhibited severe hypertensive episodes following erythropoietin infusion and required additional medication.

Schaefer (Würzburg) *responding to Stummvoll's question:* In our EPO study enclosing 15 patients, we did those measurements before and after the injection of the hormone and there was no change throughout 10 months. There never was an increase of blood pressure following the EPO injection.

Eschbach: I will share with you our experience with hypertension. In 68 patients treated in Seattle, over half of them have become hypertensive as defined by a diastolic pressure rise of 10 mmHg or more, or an increase in requirements for antihypertensive drugs. The majority of these patients had baseline hematocrits below 22, and the majority also had hypertension before beginning dialysis. Two developed malignant hypertension and of 9 anephric patients, 4 became more hypertensive. An extreme example is as follows: this individual had been anemic at least since the age of 6 and is now aged 30, being on dialysis for about 5 years. She had very mild hypertension controlled with 50 mg/day of metoproline, when she began receiving 150 U/kg, 3 ×/wk. Her diastolic blood pressure increased to 100 and after one week with a hematocrit of 35 she developed a headache and then a grand mal seizure. She had no neurological abnormalities after being admitted to the hospital.She was treated with a number of antihypertensive drugs but we could not control her blood pressure and when her pressure subsequently rose further, she developed malignant hypertension, that is, she developed eye-ground changes, intracerebral bleeding and weakness of her left arm and left leg. rhEPO therapy was discontinued and her hematocrit returned to its previous level, but despite the persistance of her severe anemia, she still requires minoxidil therapy to control her blood pressure. She is now completely recovered from all the side effects of her malignant hypertension and refuses to resume rhEPO therapy.

Bommer: I think the problem of increasing blood pressure is a multifactorial problem. It is not only related to EPO and blood viscosity. For example, some of our patients tolerated a lower body weight at the end of the dialysis, if they were treated with EPO and the anemia was improved. Such reduction of so-called dry weight during EPO treatment may counteract hypertension. On the other hand, transient virus infections can decrease body mass and if 'dry weight' is kept constant this will result in fluid overload. By this way the development of hypertension will be favored. So I think in the discussion of blood pressure changes, several factors must must be considered.

Bergström (Huddinge): Has anyone measured renin in these patients?

Samtleben: We did not in Munich, but I think the Hanover group did.

Koch: I am sorry, but we have not studied renin so far.

Contr. Nephrol., vol. 66, pp. 123–130 (Karger, Basel 1988)

In vitro and in vivo Effects of Recombinant Human Erythropoietin on Human Hemopoietic Progenitor Cells

A. Ganser[a], *M. Bergmann*[b], *B. Völkers*[a], *P. Grützmacher*[b], *D. Hoelzer*[a]

Abteilungen für [a]Hämatologie und [b]Nephrologie, Zentrum der Inneren Medizin, Johann Wolfgang Goethe-Universität, Frankfurt/M., BRD

Erythropoietin (EPO) is a circulating polypeptide hormone which serves as the main regulatory factor in red blood cell synthesis through its stimulatory activity on the erythroid precursor cells in the bone marrow to divide and differentiate into mature red blood cells [9]. Recently, the human EPO gene has been isolated and introduced into mammalian cells in culture [11, 13]. The recombinant human EPO (rhEPO) produced by these cells has been shown to be biologically and immunologically comparable to material derived from human urine [4, 12] or from sheep plasma [12]. The supply of pure, well-characterized rhEPO has allowed the start of phase I/II trials on the effect of rhEPO on the anemia in patients with chronic renal failure [5, 18, 19]. Although there are data on the effect of rhEPO on ^{59}Fe incorporation and on the immature erythroid progenitor cells BFU-E[2] [17] and the more mature CFU-E [5, 11, 13] there are only few data on either stimulatory or even suppressive effects of rhEPO on the other hemopoietic progenitor cells from the bone marrow and the peripheral blood of normal persons [2] and patients with chronic renal failure.

It therefore was the aim of the present study to analyze the effect of rhEPO on the multipotent progenitor cell CFU-GEMM, the unipotent

[1] We thank Ms. G. Euler, G. Schäfer, and S. Ströcker for excellent technical assistance.

[2] Abbreviations used: BFU-E = burst forming unit-erythroid; CFU-E = colony forming unit-erythroid; CFU-GEMM = CFU-granulocyte, erythrocyte, macrophage, megakaryocyte; CFU-GM = CFU-granulocyte, macrophage; CFU-Mk = CFU-megakaryocyte; IMDM = Iscove's modified Dulbecco's medium; Mo-CM = Mo-cell line conditioned medium.

immature erythroid progenitor cell BFU-E, the granulocytic-monocytic CFU-GM, and the megakaryocytic CFU-Mk, derived from the bone marrow of normal volunteers and of patients with chronic renal failure. Furthermore, we analyzed the in vivo effect of rhEPO on the incidence of hemopoietic progenitor cells in the peripheral blood of these patients while they were on treatment with rhEPO as part of a multicenter trial to reverse the anemia of end-stage renal failure.

Materials and Methods

Patients. Seven patients on regular dialysis treatment for terminal failure were studied prior to and during the first 8 weeks of treatment with rhEPO. They had not received any blood tranfusions in the 6 months prior to enrollment on the multicenter treatment protocol of rhEPO. Patients with a hematocrit <28% were selected for treatment with rhEPO. Three patients received 40 /kg intravenously after dialysis three times weekly, while 4 were given 120 U/kg. The incidence of hemopoietic progenitor cells in the peripheral blood of these patients was analyzed at weeks −1, 0, +1, +4, and +8 after the start of the therapy.

Cells and Cell Separation Procedure. Bone marrow cells were obtained after informed consent by aspiration from the posterior iliac crest of 6 normal healthy donors and of 3 patients undergoing hemodialysis for chronic renal failure. The low density cells were separated by Ficoll-Hypaque density centrifugation (density 1.077 g/ml). Adherent cells were removed from the low density bone marrow cells by incubation in plastic tissue culture dishes for 90 min at 37 °C. Nonadherent cells were collected by gently swirling the dishes and slowly pipetting off the culture medium containing the cells. The nonadherent low density cells were washed twice and were resuspended in IMDM. Peripheral blood mononuclear cells were obtained by venipuncture and Ficoll-Hypaque density centrifugation (density 1.077 g/ml).

Methylcellulose Culture System. Nonadherent low density bone marrow cells or low density blood mononuclear cells were cultured in a methylcellulose culture assay which allows in vitro colony formation of the multipotent hemopoietic progenitor cells CFU-GEMM and the lineage-restricted progenitor cells BFU-E, CFU-GM, and CFU-Mk [6, 7, 14]. 1×10^5 nonadherent bone marrow cells or 1×10^6 blood mononuclear cells were cultured per milliliter in IMDM containing 0.9% methylcellulose, 30% fresh frozen human plasma from a single normal donor, 50 μM 2-mercaptoethanol, 5% Mo-CM (medium conditioned for 5 days by the cytokine-producing T cell line Mo [8]). rhEPO was added at concentrations between 0.1 and 5.0 U/ml. In the experiments with peripheral blood mononuclear cells, fetal calf serum (Hyclone, Logan, Utah) and recombinant human GM-CSF (Immunex/Behringwerke, Seattle/Marburg; 5 ng/ml) [1] were substituted for human plasma and Mo-CM, respectively, while rhEPO was used at 1 U/ml. The culture plates, set up in quadruplicates, were incubated for 14 days at 37 °C and scored in situ under an inverted microscope.

Recombinant Human Erythropoietin. The rhEPO used in this study was obtained by DNA technology and has been developed jointly by Genetics Institute, Cambridge, USA, and Boehringer-Mannheim, Mannheim, FRG [11]. rhEPO is more than 98% pure and formulated in a buffered saline solution containing 1% bovine serum albumin. The specific activity of rhEPO is 173,000 U/g of hormone.

Statistical Analysis. Because of the difference in the incidence of progenitor cells in the separate bone marrow preparation the colony counts were standardized by setting the maximal value of each experiment to 100% and calculating the mean $\pm$ SEM from the separate experiments. The Wilcoxon signed rank test was used for determining the statistical significance.

Results

rhEPO supported the in vitro colony formation of BFU-E starting at 0.1 U/ml ($p < 0.05$) and reaching the maximum plateau level at 1.0 U/ml (table I). The BFU-E from the bone marrow of 3 patients with chronic renal failure were equally well supported by rhEPO as those of 6 normal controls, although slightly higher concentrations of rhEPO seemed to be required (table I). rhEPO also stimulated the in vitro growth of the multipotent progenitors CFU-GEMM from normal bone marrow, starting at 0.2 U/ml ($p < 0.05$) and reaching the plateau at concentrations of 0.5 U/ml (table II). Megakaryocytic colony formation in uremic bone marrow cultures was not increased significantly by rhEPO (table II). With regard to the granulocyte-macrophage lineage, the growth of CFU-GM from normal bone marrow was significantly decreased by 40% in the presence of 5.0 U/ml rhEPO ($p < 0.05$).

When the concentration of circulating hemopoietic progenitor cells was measured in patients undergoing therapy with rhEPO for anemia of chronic renal failure, a significant increase was found not only of the number of BFU-E but also of the number of CFU-GEMM and CFU-GM ($p < 0.05$) (fig. 1). This increase mainly occurred during the first week of therapy. In addition, the size of the colonies taken from the blood of the patients after the first week of treatment was considerably larger than at the time points before or afterwards. The increase in the number of hemopoietic progenitor cells was later followed by an increase in the hemoglobin levels (table III).

Discussion

The start of phase I and II clinical trials of rhEPO in patients with anemia of end-stage renal disease now allows to study the role of EPO in the

Table I. Effect of rhEPO on the in vitro growth of BFU-E from the bone marrow of normal persons (n = 6) and from patients on maintenance dialysis (n = 3) (mean of percentages of maximal growth ± SEM)

rhEPO U/ml	Normal	Dialysis patients
0	0 ± 0	0 ± 0
0.1	11.5 ± 14	17 ± 4
0.2	21 ± 18	39 ± 8
0.5	66 ± 16	56 ± 13
1.0	82 ± 17	56 ± 13
2.0	94 ± 4	83 ± 8
5.0	95 ± 8	96 ± 4

Table II. Effect of rhEPO on the in vitro growth of CFU-GEMM, CFU-Mk, and CFU-GM (mean of percentages of maximal growth ± SEM)

rhEPO U/ml	CFU-GEMM (n = 6)	CFU-Mk (n = 3)	CFU-GM (n = 6)
0	0 ± 0	51 ± 11	94 ± 4
0.1	16 ± 21	61 ± 10	89 ± 7
0.2	21 ± 18	49 ± 5	88 ± 10
0.5	65 ± 16	65 ± 22	93 ± 7
1.0	81 ± 12	75 ± 25	81 ± 11
2.0	84 ± 20	56 ± 18	79 ± 10
5.0	77 ± 15	68 ± 19	66 ± 14

Table III. Hemoglobin levels (g/dl) after treatment with rhEPO ($\bar{x}$ ± SEM)

rhEPO U/kg	Weeks of treatment with rhEPO				
	−1	0	+1	+4	+8
40 (n = 3)	7.7 ± 0.2	7.2 ± 0.4	7.2 ± 0.4	8.3 ± 0.6	9.3 ± 0.8
120 (n = 4)	7.7 ± 0.4	7.5 ± 0.4	7.6 ± 0.5	9.3 ± 0.4	10.2 ± 0.5

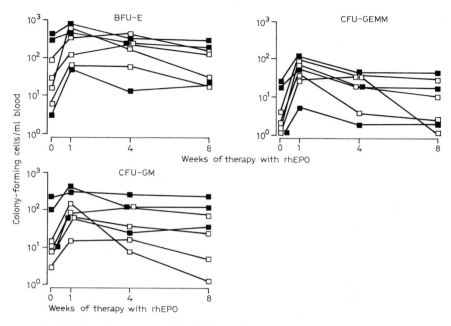

Fig. 1. Effect of treatment with rhEPO on the concentration of multipotential hemopoietic progenitors CFU-GEMM, erythroid progenitors BFU-E, and granulocyte-macrophage progenitors CFU-GM in the peripheral blood of patients with anemia of chronic
renal failure (■ = 40 U/kg; □ = 120 U/kg).

regulation of erythropoiesis in vivo [5, 18, 19]. Whereas first results indicate
the possibility that anemia is reversed in these patients by treatment with
rhEPO, demonstrating its in vivo effectiveness on erythropoiesis, the target
cells in vivo have not yet been fully characterized. The present in vitro
experiments indicate that rhEPO is an effective stimulus for human erythroid progenitor cells (BFU-E) which is in agreement with the original
biologic monitoring experiments [11, 13, 17]. In addition, they demonstrate
that rhEPO in combination with colony-stimulating factors present in
medium conditioned by the T cell line Mo (Mo-CM) [8] effectively stimulates multipotential progenitor cells to differentiate along the erythroid
lineage. Plateau levels of erythroid and multipotential colonies were stimulated in vitro by concentrations ranging from 1 to 5 U/ml.

BFU-E from patients undergoing hemodialysis for chronic renal failure
and presenting with anemia are as responsive to rhEPO in vitro as are

BFU-E from normal persons although their incidence in the bone marrow seems to be lower. This preserved responsiveness to rhEPO finds its in vivo counterpart in the increase in reticulocyte counts and hemoglobin levels after application of rhEPO in vivo [5, 18, 19].

To determine whether rhEPO promoted megakaryocytic differentiation, we analyzed the effect of rhEPO on megakaryocytic colony formation. In contrast to data obtained with murine cells [3] but in agreement with previously reported data with human bone marrow cells [2, 15], we were unable to find any stimulatory activity of rhEPO on megakaryocytic colony formation in the presence of optimal concentrations of Mo-CM. rhEPO therefore seems not to influence megakaryopoiesis at the progenitor cell level, but to act at a later stage, possibly increasing the DNA content of the megakaryocytes [10]. Similar observations have recently been reported in a serum-free culture system using mouse spleen cells [12, 15].

The granulocyte-macrophage colony formation was significantly inhibited at the higher concentrations of EPO used which might be due to the induction of erythroid differentiation in multipotent progenitor cells leading to a decrease in the number of granulocytic-monocytic colonies.

When rhEPO was given three times weekly to the patients with chronic renal failure dosages between 40 and 120 U/kg, the concentrations of BFU-E, CFU-GEMM, and CFU-GM in the peripheral blood significantly increased during the first week of therapy followed by a slight decrease during the subsequent weeks. The underlying physiological mechanisms responsible for these changes remain unclear, but direct and indirect stimulation of the progenitor cells by rhEPO are feasible.

The increase in the size of the colonies grown in vitro which was especially prominent after the first week of therapy further supports the hypothesis that the hemopoietic progenitor cells are activated in vivo by treatment with rhEPO. While the activation of erythroid progenitors by rhEPO, which was followed by an increase in hemoglobin levels, was an expected observation, the number of CFU-GM also increased during in vivo application of rhEPO pointing to the complexity of the regulation of hemopoiesis which not always allows a prediction of in vivo findings from in vitro observations.

In conclusion, rhEPO is an effective stimulus of erythroid proliferation and differentiation both in vitro and in vivo in patients with anemia of chronic renal failure. Further studies in vitro and in vivo have to clarify its potential role in the treatment of other disorders of erythropoiesis.

References

1 Cantrell, M. T.; Anderson, D.; Cerretti, D. P.; Price, V.; McKereghan, K.; Tushinski, R. R.; Mochizuki, D. Y.; Larsen, A.; Grabstein, K.; Gillis, S.; Cosman, D.: Cloning, sequence, and expression of a human granulocyte/macrophage colony-stimulating factor. Proc. natn. Acad. Sci. USA *82:* 6250–6254 (1985).

2 Dessypris, E. N.; Gleaton, J. H.; Armstrong, O. L.: Effect of human recombinant erythropoietin on human marrow megakaryocyte colony formation in vitro. Br. J. Haemat. *65:* 265–269 (1987).

3 Dukes, P. P.; Egrie, J. C.; Strickland, T. W.; Browne, J. K.; Lin, F. K.: Megakaryocyte colony stimulating activity of recombinant human and monkey erythropoietin; in Levine, Williams, Levine, Evatt, Megakaryocyte development and function, pp. 105–109 (Liss, New York, 1986).

4 Egrie, J. C.; Strickland, T. W.; Lane, J.; Aoki, K.; Cohen, A. M.; Smalling, R.; Trail, G.; Lin, F. K.; Browne, J. K.; Hines, D. K.: Characterization and biological effects of recombinant human erythropoietin. Immunobiology *172:* 213–224 (1986).

5 Eschbach, J. W.; Egrie, J. C.; Downing, M. R.; Browne, J. K.; Adamson, J. W.: Correction of anemia of end-stage renal disease with recombinant human erythropoietin: results of a combined phase I and II clinical trial. New Engl. J. Med. *316:* 73–78 (1987).

6 Fauser, A. A.; Messner, H. A.: Granuloerythropoietic colonies in human bone marrow, peripheral blood and cord blood. Blood *52:* 1243–1248 (1978).

7 Ganser, A.; Elstner, E.; Hoelzer, D.: Megakaryocytic cells in mixed haemopoietic colonies (CFU-GEMM) from the peripheral blood of normal individuals. Br. J. Haemat. *59:* 627–633 (1985).

8 Golde, D. W.; Quan, S. G.; Cline, M. J.: Human T lymphocyte cell line producing colony-stimulating activity. Blood *52:* 1068–1072.

9 Graber, S. E.; Krantz, S. B.: Erythropoietin and the control of red blood cell production. A. Rev. Med. *29:* 51–66 (1978).

10 Ishibashi, T.; Koziol, J. A.; Burstein, S. A.: Human recombinant erythropoietin promotes differentiation of murine megakaryocytes in vitro. J. clin. Invest. *79:* 286–289 (1987).

11 Jacobs, K.; Shoemaker, C.; Rudersdorf, R.; Neill, S. D.; Kaufman, R. J.; Mufson, A.; Seehra, J.; Jones, S. S.; Hewick, R.; Fritsch, E. F.; Kawakita, M.; Shimizu, T.; Miyake, T.: Isolation and characterization of genome and cDNA clones of human erythropoietin. Nature, Lond. *313:* 306–310 (1985).

12 Koike, K.; Shimizu, T.; Miyake, T.; Ihle, J. N.; Ogawa, M.: Hemopoietic colony formation by mouse spleen cells in serum-free culture supported by purified erythropoietin and/or interleukin 3; in Levine, Williams, Levine, Evatt, Megakaryocyte development and function, pp. 33–49 (Liss, New York, 1986).

13 Lin, F. K.; Suggs, S.; Lin, C. H.; et al.: Cloning and expression of the human erythropoietin gene. Proc. natn. Acad. Sci. USA *82:* 7580–7584 (1985).

14 Messner, H. A.; Jamal, N.: Izaguirre, C.: The growth of large megakaryocyte colonies from human bone marrow. J. cell. Physiol. *1:* suppl., pp. 45–51 (1982).

15 Mizoguchi, H.; Fujiwara, Y.; Sasaki, R.; Chiba, H.: The effect of interleukin-3 and erythropoietin on murine megakaryocyte colony formation; in Levine, Williams,

Levine, Evatt, Megakaryocyte development and function, pp. 111–115 (Liss, New York 1986).

16   Sawada, K.; Krantz, S. B.; Kans, J. S.; Dessypris, E. N.; Sawyer, S.; Glick, A. D.; Civin, C. I.: Purification of human erythroid colony forming units and demonstration of specific binding of erythropoietin. J. clin. Invest. *80:* 357–366 (1987).

17   Sieff, C. A.; Emerson, S. G.; Mufson, A.; Gesner, T. G.; Nathan, D. G.: Dependence of highly enriched human bone marrow progenitors on hemopoietic growth factors and their response to recombinant erythropoietin. J. clin. Invest. *77:* 74–81 (1986).

18   Winearls, C. G.; Oliver, D. O.; Pippard, M. J.; Reid, C.; Downing, M. R.; Cotes, P. M.: Effect of human erythropoietin derived from recombinant DNAS on the anaemia of patients maintained by chronic haemodialysis. Lancet *ii:* 1175–1178 (1986).

19   Zins, B.; Drüeke, T.; Zingraff, J.: Bererhi, L.; Kreis, H.: Naret, C.; Delors, S.; Castaigne, J. P.; Peterlongo, F.; Casadevall, N.; Varet, B.: Erythropoietin treatment in anaemic patients on haemodialysis. Lancet *ii:* 1329 (1986).

Dr. A. Ganser, Abteilung für Hämatologie, Zentrum der Inneren Medizin, Klinikum der Johann Wolfgang Goethe Universität, Theodor-Stern-Kai 7, D-6000 Frankfurt 70 (FRG)

Discussion

Müller-Wiefel: How do you explain the low response of the erythroid progenitor cells of the uremic patients? From all we heard and talked about today I believe this phenomenon should not be observed.

Ganser: One reason, of course, could be that the number of patients I showed to you here are not very large and it could be a statistical problem. On the other hand, there is no doubt that the incidence of the progenitor cells in the bone marrow of these patients is lower than normal. Of course, we have to take into account that we are not working with pure stem cell suspensions. The data on the colony counts here, in addition, represents the growth in culture, and this, of course, is influenced by various other factors too. There are many cells, like macrophages and T cells, that can be activated and can exert some suppressive effects. I could imagine that, for instance, after dialysis you can have stimulation of T suppressor cells which exert a suppressive action on the hemopoietic progenitor cells.

Koch: How do you reconcile your data with the observed increase in thrombocytes seen in the multicentre trial?

Ganser: As I mentioned before (I hoped it became clear), investigators reporting an effect of erythropoietin on megakaryocytic progenitor cells worked in a system with suboptimal concentrations of CSF. Otherwise there would have been no further stimulation of the colony growth by erythropoietin. What we did in our system, was that we always have used maximum stimulation by GM-CSF and by interleukin 3. Thus, erythropoietin could actually not exert any further stimulatory effects in our system.

Contr. Nephrol., vol. 66, pp. 131–138 (Karger, Basel 1988)

Treatment of Polytransfused Hemodialysis Patients with Recombinant Human Erythropoietin

J. Bommer, W. Huber, G. Tewes, E. Ritz, S. von Wedel, S. Küppers, T. Weinreich, G. Bommer

Medizinische Universitätsklinik, Heidelberg, und Rehabilitationszentrum, Heidelberg-Wieblingen, BRD

Inappropriately low erythropoietin (EPO) levels seem to be the major cause, among other factors, of anemia in chronic hemodialysis patients. Particularly in binephrectomized patients, despite adequate hemodialysis, severe anemia may often necessitate repeated blood tranfusions which may further suppress residual EPO production. Furthermore, blood transfusions carry the risks of iron overload, i. e. hemosiderosis, and of transfer of infectious diseases, e.g. non-A, non-B hepatitis, cytomegalo or HIV virus infection.

Consequently, the availability of recombinant human erythropoietin (rhEPO) opens the perspective that in the future blood transfusion may be avoided altogether in chronic hemodialysis patients. Recent studies in both non-transfused and polytransfused dialysis patients showed that serum hemoglobin can be raised by a three times weekly administration of rhEPO after hemodialysis [1–3]. However, several points needed to be clarified, e. g. optimal dose, optimal frequency of application and exhaustive analysis of potential side effects. The following study on rhEPO treatment was performed to address these issues.

Patients and Methods

Nine polytransfused patients (5 males, 4 females) requiring 5–20 units of packed erythrocytes during the preceding 12 months were treated with rhEPO. The mean age was 40.4 ± 16.7 (SD) years. The mean duration of dialysis was 95 ± 60 months; all patients were on dialysis for more than 2 years. All patients were dialyzed three times per week for 5 h using AB Gambro AK 10 or Drake Willock DWS 4035 machines and as plate dialyzers AB Gambro Lundia N5 or hollow-fiber dialyzers AB Gambro 1.8 M or MTS C 1.3 (Fresenius Co.).

All patients were normotensive without antihypertensive medication. One patient was consistently hypotensive with systolic blood pressure constantly below 100 mm Hg. Hemolysis, gastrointestinal bleeding, aluminum intoxication, deficiency of vitamin B_{12} and folic acid were excluded by appropriate measurements. Patients did not have chronic infection, immunosuppressive therapy, histories of drug or alcohol abuse or severe hyperparathyroidism.

Protocol

Baseline laboratory values were collected during 8–12 weeks prior to the last blood transfusion. Subsequently, patients received a constant dose of three times weekly 100 U rhEPO/kg body weight (Cilag-Ortho-Amgen Co., Alsbach-Hähnlein). The first infusion was given immediately following the last blood transfusion. The following laboratory examinations were performed: three times per week hematological status and once weekly serum chemistry, i. e. transaminases, electrolytes, creatinine, iron, coagulation profile; ferritin, transferrin and haptoglobin were measured monthly. The following methods were used: blood cells by Coulter counter; serum chemistry by multichannel autoanalyzer; reticulocytes and differential counts manually; ferritin by radioimmunoassay; transferrin by immunodiffusion (Partigen). To correct for the influence of anemia, reticulocyte counts were given as absolute reticulocyte counts (% reticulocytes × erythrocyte count). Before and after dialysis as well as half an hour after rhEPO injection, blood pressure, heart rate and body temperature were monitored. Hollow-fiber clotting was evaluated by staff members with a preestablished score system.

All data are given as mean ± SD.

Results

Within 1 week after the start of rhEPO treatment, reticulocyte counts increased and reached a maximum after 3 weeks (initial: $30.7 \pm 13.2 \times 10^9/l$; maximum: $103 \pm 41.8 \times 10^9/l$) (table I). Hematocrit continued to decrease during the first 2 weeks in most of the patients (fig. 1). During the following weeks, hematocrit levels increased in all patients. After 2–3 months, hemoglobin had increased from 5.9 ± 0.85 g/dl (baseline) to 11.2 ± 0.8 g/dl. No further transfusions were required under rhEPO in any patient. Thrombocyte counts increased from $157 \pm 42.1 \times 10^9/l$ to $191 \pm 51.1 \times 10^9/l$. In 2 of the 9 patients, no increase of thrombocyte counts was found.

In parallel with the increase in erythropoiesis, a decrease in serum ferritin levels was noted. Because of excessive serum ferritin levels at the start of the study, iron supplementation was not considered to be necessary in any of the patients. Under rhEPO treatment, major side effects were not observed, but

Table I. rhEPO treatment in polytransfused dialysis patients

	Pretreatment period	End of dose-finding period	Long-term follow-up period
Hemoglobin, g/dl	5.9 ± 0.85	11.2 ± 0.8	10.5 ± 0.9
Erythrocytes, 10^{12}/l	1.83 ± 0.34	3.45 ± 0.38	3.2 ± 0.22
Abs. reticulocytes, 10^9/l	30.7 ± 13.2	100.3 ± 41.8	57.6 ± 21.6
Platelets, 10^9/l	156.9 ± 42.1	190.6 ± 51.1	169 ± 41

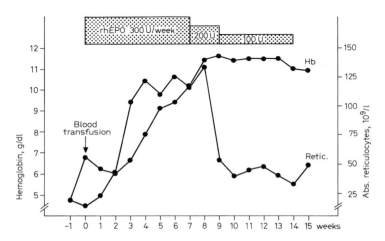

Fig. 1. rhEPO treatment in patient R.W. Doses given in U/kg/week.

an increase of mean predialysis systolic blood pressure was found in all patients (118 ± 23 mm Hg before and 130 ± 27 mm Hg during rhEPO therapy).

Discussion

The present study documents an increase of hemoglobin during treatment with 100 U rhEPO/kg three times per week in dialysis patients. This result is in good agreement with previous reports [1–5].

In our anemic polytransfused dialysis patients without overt bleeding, hemoglobin continued to decrease during the first 2 weeks of the study, but further blood transfusions were no longer required. A continuous rise in hemoglobin was observed in all patients by the third week of rhEPO treatment (fig. 1). The dose of 100 U rhEPO/kg three times weekly seems to be sufficient to raise hemoglobin levels to more than 10 g/dl in polytransfused patients after treatment for 2–3 months.

Similar rhEPO doses have previously also been shown to be effective in nontransfused dialysis patients [3, 6], indicating that in polytransfused but anemic patients the bone marrow has not become hyporesponsive to EPO. The dose-dependent increase of reticulocyte counts in polytransfused patients was quantitatively comparable with the finding in nontransfused anemic dialysis patients [3].

When the patients had reached a hemoglobin level exceeding 10 g/dl for 1 week, the dose of rhEPO was reduced. Within 1 week, such reduction of rhEPO was followed by a fall in reticulocyte counts.

Thrombocyte counts increased in 7/9 of our polytransfused patients. The increase was dose dependent: thrombocyte counts decreased when the dose of rhEPO was reduced at the end of the study. The increase in thrombocyte counts by 22% was comparable in magnitude with our previous observations in nontransfused dialysis patients [3, 5]. Further confirming our previous studies, no change of leukocyte counts was found and several laboratory parameters remained unchanged, i. e. transaminases, bilirubin, bicarbonate, electrolytes. Serum potassium levels showed erratic upward swings in some patients. However, patients had very intensely been instructed about potential risks of hyperkalemia and hyperphosphatemia under rhEPO treatment, and were presumably sticking to dietary restrictions and oral phosphate binders, respectively.

As expected, serum ferritin levels decreased under rhEPO treatment. At least over 3 months a modest decrease of serum ferritin levels was observed in those patients who had excessive initial serum ferritin levels, i. e. >2,000 µg/l. In patients with lower starting serum ferritin levels, the decrease was more readily demonstrable, e. g. from a median starting level of 1,000 to 855 µg/l. Treatment with rhEPO does not only offer the benefit to raise hematocrit, but may also be indicated to reverse hemosiderosis and iron overload in polytransfused patients. Whether or not rhEPO treatment can be combined with venesection in patients with iron overload, will require further consideration and study.

In previous studies, a flu-like syndrome and other mild side effects were observed after rhEPO injections. Apparently, the symptoms were more frequent when the drug was injected rapidly. In the present study, rhEPO was slowly infused over 2–3 min. Under these conditions, patients did not report any discomfort. A moderate, but consistent increase in blood pressure in parallel with the rise in hematocrit was found in all patients, but marked hypertension or hypertensive crises were not noted. As in previous studies, the rise in blood pressure followed the rise in hematocrit and seems not to be a direct effect of rhEPO.

References

1   Winearls, C. G.; Oliver, D. O.; Pippard, M. J.; Reid, C.; Downing, M. R.; Cotes, P. M.: Effects of human erythropoietin derived from recombinant DNA on the anemia of patients maintained by chronic hemodialysis. Lancet *ii:* 1175–1177 (1986).
2   Eschbach, J. W.; Egrie, J. C.; Downing, M. R.; Browne, J. K.; Adamson, J. W.: Correction of the anemia of end-stage renal disease with recombinant human erythropoietin. New Engl. J. Med. *316:* 73–78 (1987).
3   Bommer, J.; Alexiou, C.; Müller-Bühl, U.; Eifert, J.; Ritz, E.: Recombinant human erythropoietin therapy in haemodialysis patients – dose determination and clinical experience. Nephrol. Dial. Transplant. *2:* 238–242 (1987).
4   Zins, B.; Drüeke, T.; Zingraff, J.; Bererhi, L.; Kreis, H.; Naret, C.; Delors, S.; Castaigne, J. P.; Peterlongo, F.; Casadevall, N.; Varet, B.: Erythropoietin treatment in anaemic patients on haemodialysis (letter). Lancet *ii:* 1329 (1986).
5   Bommer, J.; Müller-Bühl, E.; Ritz, E.; Eifert, J.: Recombinant human erythropoietin in anaemic patients on haemodialysis (letter). Lancet *ii:* 392 (1987).
6   Stutz, B.; Rhyner, K.; Vögtli, J.; Binswanger, U.: Erfolgreiche Behandlung der Anämie bei Hämodialyse-Patienten mit rekombiniertem humanem Erythropoietin. Schweiz. med. Wschr. *117:* 1397–1402 (1987).

Prof. Dr. J. Bommer, Klinikum der Universität, Bergheimerstrasse 58, D-6900 Heidelberg 1 (FRG)

Discussion

Müller-Wiefel: Maybe I did not catch it, but what was the reason for the transfusion dependency of your patients? You excluded nearly every mechanism which might have been possible. Were the patients bilaterally nephrectomised?

Bommer: In patients who were on long-term hemodialysis, particularly in patients who have a dialysis time of more than 10 years, you can observe a certain number of patients who require blood transfusion. And if such patients have started to be transfused, often they have a continuous requirement of blood transfusion over years. It is not possible to stop transfusion therapy.

Kühn: What was the course of the corrected reticulocyte counts?

Bommer: The corrected reticulocyte counts paralleled the absolute reticulocyte counts. For the corrected reticulocyte count, you multiply the reticulocyte count with the current hematocrit and divide the value by 45. For the absolute reticulocyte count, you multiply the reticulocyte count with the erythrocyte count. Since the erythrocyte count parallels the hematocrit, both calculations imply the same correction. Therefore, you can compare the time course of corrected reticulocyte counts with that of absolute reticulocyte counts.

Nattermann: What was your indication for blood transfusion? Was it just the feeling of the patient or was it a certain hemoglobin level?

Bommer: I cannot give you a general answer; there are different indications. For example, there is an old lady who suffers from severe hemosiderosis. We suspect that she has also hemosiderosis of the myocardium. This lady required blood transfusion because she got angina pectoris and dyspnea if the hematocrit levels decreased below 22%. In other patients, hematocrit fell to less than 18 or 17% before they were transfused. There was no absolute level of hematocrit at which blood transfusions were necessary. We have also 4 rather young people who required blood transfusion. All patients had clinical symptoms which required the transfusion therapy.

Koch: Do you think that the response of hematocrit in these iron-overloaded patients was faster than in patients without iron overload?

Bommer: If we compare these patients with a group of patients without iron overload, treated with 120 U rhEPO/kg body weight, we found a rather comparable response of hematocrit to rhEPO treatment. The response of hematocrit varied markedly from patient to patient, but in the mean, after 8 weeks in most patients hematocrit levels were corrected. That may take 1 week longer in polytransfused iron-overloaded patients, because of the decrease of hematocrit during the first or second week after transfusion. However, the response of hematocrit was not markedly different in patients with and without iron overload.

Bergström (Huddinge): Dr. Bommer, you mentioned that you are using a platelet inhibitor in these studies. I would like to ask you which platelet inhibitor you are using? Is this something which you recommend other groups to do also?

Bommer: We used acetylsalicylate and we have good experiences. In our opinion, it is very useful. If the hematocrit increased to more than 27%, we treated most patients with platelet inhibitors.

Bergström: Which dosage?

Bommer: Many years ago we used a high dose of 5 g per day, but now we sometimes use doses of lower than 1 g per week.

Winearls (London): Can you tell us why you are using a platelet inhibitor?

Bommer: That is a very difficult question. We observed fistula clotting during a previous study of rhEPO treatment in patients who had no transfusion. We have the impression that the fistula clotting was less frequent if the patients were treated with platelet inhibitors. Ten years ago, Prof. Andrassy of our group published a randomized prospective study of patients with and without platelet inhibitor therapy after fistula surgery. Fistula clotting was less frequent in patients with platelet inhibitors. We have the impression that frequency of fistula clotting can be reduced by the application of platelet inhibitors.

Winearls: Do you mean you put the rest of your patients on platelet inhibitors?

Bommer: Hemodialysis patients with hematocrit levels between 20 and 25% and well functioning arteriovenous fistulae were not treated with platelet inhibitors. But, for example, patients with Gore-Tex protheses were all treated with platelet inhibitors.

Winearls: My second point concerns the ferritin levels in the polytransfused patients. We have noticed the same transient fall in ferritins. In those patients who are heavily transfused and have high ferritins there is a transient fall at the time of maximal response. When the patients reach their maintenance, the ferritin returns to near the pretreatment levels. Does this reflect rapid mobilisation of iron during rapid response? It is going to take quite a long time to mobilise all the iron in these patients. To return to your point about whether you can venesect these patients: it would actually be quite interesting to see, if you did aggressively venesect them, whether the hemoglobins fell. Because if you take the example of hemochromatosis you can actually make patients have iron-deficient erythropoiesis despite the fact that they are iron-loaded. So we will have to wait and see. Do you have ferritin levels later on?

Bommer: We now have experience in rhEPO treatment of 6 months and no more in polytransfused patients. So I cannot give you an answer for the long-term effects on serum ferritin levels.

Winearls: We can ask Dr. Eschbach – he has got a lot of polytransfused patients – whether he has noticed a continued fall in the ferritin or whether they have come back to baseline.

Eschbach: In contrast to Dr. Winearl's experience, the serum ferritin levels in our patients have continued to decrease with rhEPO treatment. After a year of treatment the highest ferritin levels, in general, are reduced in half. When rhEPO treatment is stopped the ferritin levels do increase, but none return to previous baselines. In reference to Prof. Koch's question: the reason the polytransfused patients do so well with rhEPO therapy, in contrast to other patients, is that they have plenty of iron. If one examines the response in other patients, many of them don't have as rapid a rise in hematocrit levels because they may develop iron deficiency during acute rhEPO therapy.

Bommer: I think that is a very important point. The iron status is a determining factor for the hematocrit response after EPO therapy. May I ask you a question, Dr. Eschbach: Have you measured the liver density by computer tomography in such patients with iron overload? Sometimes, we found an increased density by liver scan, and even if this is a crude parameter of iron overload in these patients, it would be interesting to perform follow-up studies.

Eschbach: No we have not. The only analogy relates to one of our patients who has marked hepatosplenomegaly and thrombocytopenia as the result of transfusion-induced iron overload. After 9 months of treatment his spleen is now smaller by physical examination.

Wizemann (Giessen): The lady you mentioned who suffered from myocardial iron overload, did she improve with respect to her myocardial function?

Bommer: It is difficult to evaluate improvement of myocardial function in such patients with increasing hematocrit after EPO treatment. The physical fitness of this patient was much better but we found no marked change by echocardiography. I think 6 months is too short to expect a marked decrease of hemosiderosis of the myocardium in such a patient. We have to control the patient perhaps after 1 year. At the moment, we have no data clearly indicating an improvement of myocardial function.

Wizemann: Did she also have a rise in blood pressure?

Bommer: There was an increase of the systolic blood pressure in this patient, but that is a common finding. This patient was not hypotensive during the time before the EPO treatment and we cannot conclude that cardiac insufficiency results in hypotensive blood pressure in this patient.

Wizemann: You mentioned that this patient had angina pectoris. Could you manage her better during EPO than with the polytransfusions?

Bommer: The angina was mostly related to the hematocrit level. The hematocrit is now high so angina has disappeared.

Contr. Nephrol., vol. 66, pp. 139–148 (Karger, Basel 1988)

Treatment of a Seven-Year-Old Child with End-Stage Renal Disease and Hemosiderosis by Recombinant Human Erythropoietin

R. Burghard[a], *J. Leititis*[a], *R. Pallacks*[a], *P. Scigalla*[b], *M. Brandis*[a]

[a]Zentrum für Kinderheilkunde der Philipps-Universität, Marburg, und
[b]Boehringer Mannheim GmbH, Mannheim, BRD

Anemia is an almost invariable feature of chronic renal failure and is particularly severe in children treated by a long-term maintenance hemodialysis. Most of these patients require blood transfusions with the attendant risks of hepatitis, sensitization to histocompatibility antigens and iron overload. In addition, anemia may contribute considerably to decreased activity and well-being. Anemia is suspected to be an important factor for growth retardation of children with end-stage renal disease; however, the relationship between renal anemia and somatic growth is not well defined [6].

An increasing number of reports demonstrate that the anemia of end-stage renal disease is principally reversible by recombinant human erythropoietin (rhEPO) in adults [1–5, 8–10]. In children, however, the potential benefits and side-effects of rhEPO have not been studied so far in clinical trials. Therefore, a first report on the treatment of a 7-year-old child receiving rhEPO for life-threatening complications from severe secondary hemochromatosis is presented.

Case Report

The underlying cause of end-stage renal disease was a hemolytic-uremic syndrome at the age of 6 years, leading to maintenance hemodialysis (12 h weekly) in November 1985. The clinical course was complicated by severe hypertension requiring treatment with propranolol, dihydralazine, nifedipine and captopril in high dosages. A kidney transplantation from a cadaveric donor was performed in June 1986. 15 days later, the graft had to be removed after a transplant biopsy which was followed by a unappeasable hemorrhage from the site of biopsy into the retro- and intraperitoneal space. During the postoperative period disseminated intravascular coagulation developed and transfusions of a total amount of 27 units of packed red cells (PRC) and 10 units of thrombocyte concentrate were necessary.

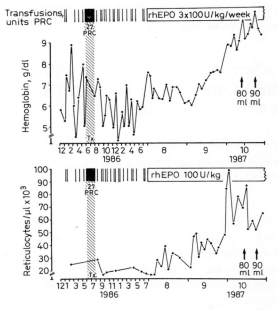

Fig. 1. Effect of rhEPO on erythropoiesis (hemoglobin and reticulocytes). Arrows indicate blood loss. Tx = Transplantation.

Two months later the patient experienced 92% cytotoxic antibodies and showed clinical and laboratory signs of severe secondary hemochromatosis, affecting predominantly the skin, liver and heart. Serum ferritin levels were already elevated before transplantation (744 µg/l) but excessively increased after graft removal (5,500 µg/l). Under regular hemodialysis, the patient continued to require 1.4 units PRC per month and serum ferritin levels were increased to a maximum of 7,100 µg/l.

In June 1987, an atrioventricular block led to cardiac arrest and cardiopulmonary resuscitation. A pacemaker was inserted because of persisting bradyarrythmias, probably due to heart hemochromatosis. Serum ferritin levels at that time ranged between 5,700 and 7,100 µg/l. Two months later, rhEPO treatment was instituted after informed parental consent to participation in this experimental clinical trial.

Study Protocol for rhEPO Treatment

Lyophilizated rhEPO (Boehringer, Mannheim), 100 U/kg, was administered three times weekly as an intravenous short-time infusion (20 min) at the end of each routine dialysis treatment. Temperature, blood pressure, pulse, and respiration rates were recorded 30–60 min after infusion of rhEPO. Blood counts were done with a Coulter counter and reticulocytes were counted by standard methods three times a week before hemodialysis. A

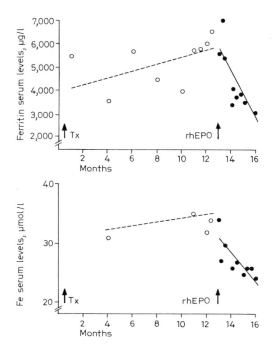

Fig. 2. Serum ferritin and serum iron before (○) and after (●) rhEPO treatment.
Tx = Transplantation.

biochemical serum profile (creatinine, BUN, potassium, phosphorus) including information on iron status (ferritin, iron, transferrin) was performed weekly.

Iron elimination by venesection was started when hemoglobin levels were >10 g/dl
and hematocrit was >30%. The blood volume removed after hemodialysis corresponded to
5% of the estimated total blood volume and ranged between 80 and 90 ml each. Iron
elimination therapy aimed at serum ferritin levels <150 µg/l.

Results

The effect of rhEPO treatment on hemoglobin levels and reticulocyte
count is delineated in figure 1. Reticulocytes increased 15 days after institution of rhEPO and hemoglobin levels stabilized at a value of 6.5 g/dl. No
further transfusions were required, while rhEPO treatment was carried out.
A steady increase of hemoglobin concentration was observed after 6 weeks
of therapy and two venesections were realized after 10 and 12 weeks.

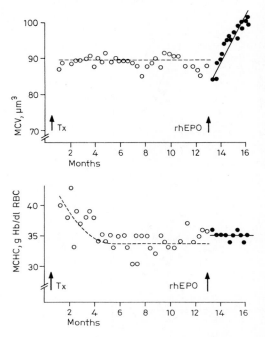

Fig. 3. MCV and MCHC before (○) and after (●) rhEPO treatment. Tx = Transplantation.

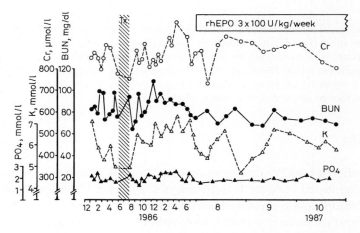

Fig. 4. Serum concentrations of creatinine (Cr), urea (BUN), potassium (K), and phosphorus (PO_4) before and during rhEPO treatment. Tx = Transplantation.

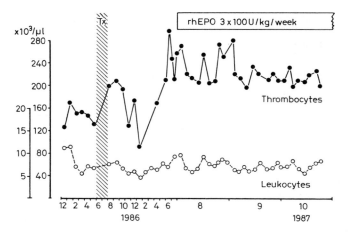

Fig. 5. Platelet and leukocyte count before and during rhEPO treatment. Tx = Transplantation.

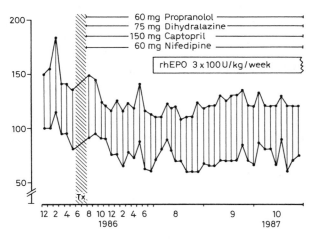

Fig. 6. Blood pressure and antihypertensive drugs before and during rhEPO treatment. Tx = Transplantation.

Serum ferritin and serum iron levels declined significantly during the first 3 months after rhEPO treatment and iron elimination therapy (fig. 2). Mean corpuscular erythrocyte volume (MCV) was rather constant throughout regular hemodialysis before rhEPO treatment, but showed a steep increment after rhEPO treatment whereas mean corpuscular hemoglobin

Table I. Clinical and laboratory data 3 months before and after treatment with rhEPO

	Before	After
Transfusions, U/month	1.4	0
Hb, g/dl	5.8 (5.5–6.2)	7.5 (6.8–8.5)
Hct, %	17 (16–18)	22 (19–24)
Reticulocytes/µl × 10^3	21.3 (16.6–28.0)	38.1 (29.6–46.2)
Ferritin, µg/l × 10^3	5.7 (5.6–5.9)	3.6 (3.5–4.3)
Fe, µmol/l	33 (32–34)	27 (26–27)
MCV	86 (85–88)	93 (91–95)
Thrombocytes/µl × 10^3	213 (210–246)	221 (206–230)

Medians, 95% confidence limits in parentheses.

concentration (MCHC) was unaffected (fig. 3). No severe side effects have been noted so far. Predialytic creatinine, potassium and phosphorus levels remained constant and modalities of dialysis treatment – including heparinization – were not changed during rhEPO treatment (fig. 4). Thrombocytes tended to increase slightly but were within the normal range (fig. 5). Maximal platelet count after rhEPO treatment was 280,000/µl compared to 286,000/µl in the pretreatment period. Total leukocyte count remained completely unchanged. Blood pressure was only poorly controlled under maximal antihypertensive therapy irrespective of rhEPO administration; rhEPO did not increase blood pressure above baseline values and no variation of antihypertensive drugs or dose adjustment were required (fig. 6).

In table I the main clinical and laboratory features comparing the 3-month period before and after rhEPO treatment are summarized.

Discussion

Hitherto, clinical trials to correct anemia of end-stage renal disease by treatment with rhEPO have only been reported in adult patients [1–5, 8–10]. From these studies it is evident that rhEPO is effective in a dose-dependent manner and can restore the hemoglobin levels and the hematocrit to normal in many patients. Along with the stimulation of erythropoiesis, the need for transfusions is generally decreased or eliminated during rhEPO treatment [5, 9]. These findings may be of special importance to pediatric patients in whom severe anemia may contribute not only to decreased well-being but also to decreased caloric intake and – directly or indirectly – to growth delay. However, no broad experience exists so far in rhEPO treatment during childhood.

The possibility that treatment with rhEPO combined with venesection may permit the correction of serious iron overload in patients with end-stage renal disease [5, 9] justified an experiment trial of rhEPO treatment in a child with severe complications from secondary hemochromatosis. A three times weekly dose regimen of 100 U/kg rhEPO resulted in a subsequent stimulation of erythropoiesis. The hemoglobin target value (10 g/dl) for envisioned iron elimination therapy was reached after 10 weeks and no further transfusions were required. Serum ferritin levels decreased markedly during the first 3 months of follow-up, consistent with the exhaustion of iron stores. Concomitantly MCV increased after initiation of rhEPO treatment. These findings probably represent an internal shift of iron from reticuloendothelial or parenchymal sites to newly formed red cells.

From adult studies there is evidence that raising the hemoglobin concentration and blood viscosity enhances potential risks which may be relevant especially in patients prone to accelerated vascular disease [9]. In our young patient, no side effects that could be related directly or indirectly to rhEPO were observed during the first 3 months of treatment.

A significant increase in blood pressure has been reported especially in previously hypertensive adult patients [4]. Blood pressure was poorly controlled in our patient before rhEPO administration, but was not further elevated above baseline values during treatment.

It has been suggested that decreasing dialyzer clearances combined with increased well-being and appetite as hematocrit rises, may lead to a state of underdialysis [5]. The metabolic situation, however, was not deteriorated in our patient despite unchanged dialysis modalities. A slight but clinically insignificant increase of platelet count probably reflects a stimulative effect of rhEPO on megakaryopoiesis [2, 3, 8, 11].

The benefits of rhEPO treatment in this preliminary report on a single child are an improvement in patient well-being and elimination of the need for blood transfusions. Although no direct or indirect side effects were noted during 3 months of treatment, further careful observation is required to assess the individual adaptation mechanisms of the previously anemic patient to an increasing red cell mass and blood viscosity. The long-term effects of near-normal hemoglobin concentrations from maintenance rhEPO therapy remain to be evaluated by prospective clinical trials in children.

References

1 Akizawa, T.; Kochikawa, S.; Takaku, F.; Urabe, A.; Akiyama, N.; Otsubu, O.; Mimura, N.; Nihei, H.; Kawaguchi, Y.; Ota, K.; Kubo, K.: Clinical effect of recombinant human erythropoietin (r-hu EPO) on anemia associated with chronic renal failure. Multi-center cooperative study in Japan. Artif. Organs *11:* 301 (1987).

2 Bommer, J.; Müller-Bühl, E.; Rith, E.; Eifert, J.: Recombinant erythropoietin in anemic patients on hemodialysis. Lancet *i:* 392 (1987).

3 Bommer, J., Ritz, E.; Alexiu, C.; Eifert, J.: R-hu EPO therapy in anemic dialysis patients. Abstr. Xth Int. Congr. Nephrol., London (1987).

4 Casati, S.; Passerini, P.; Graziani, G.; Moia, M.; Della Valle, P.; Mannucci, P. M.; Ponticelli, C.: Human recombinant erythropoietin corrects anemia and bleeding tendency in hemodialysis patients. Abstr. Xth Int. Congr. Nephrol., London 1987.

5 Eschbach, J. W.; Egrie, J. C.; Downing, M. R.; Browne, J. K.; Adamson, J. W.: Correction of the anemia of end-stage renal disease with recombinant human erythropoietin. New Engl. J. Med. *316:* 73–78 (1987).

6 Holliday, M. A.: Growth retardation in children with renal disease; in Edelmann, Pediatric kidney disease, pp. 331–341 (Little, Brown, Boston 1978).

7 Schaefer, R. M.; Kuerner, B.; Zech, M.; Heidland, A.: Treatment of the anemia of patients maintained by hemodialysis with recombinant human erythropoietin. Artif. Organs *11:* 307 (1987).

8 Stutz, B.; Rhyner, K.; Vögtli, J.; Binswanger, U.: Erfolgreiche Behandlung der Anämie bei Hämodialyse-Patienten mit rekombiniertem humanem Erythropoietin. Schweiz. med. Wschr. *117:* 1397–1402 (1987).

9 Winearls, C. G.; Oliver, D. O.; Pippard, M. J.; Reid, C.; Downing, M. R.; Cotes, P. M.: Effect of human erythropoietin derived from recombinant DNA on the anaemia of patients maintained by chronic haemodialysis. Lancet *ii:* 1175–1178 (1986).

10 Winearls, C. G.; Cotes, P. M; Pippard, M.; Ried, C.; Oliver, D. O.: Correction of anaemia in haemodialysis patients with recombinant erythropoietin – follow-up and results of pharmacokinetic, ferrokinetic and bone marrow culture studies. Abstr. Xth Int. Congr. Nephrol., London 1987.

11 Toshiyuki, I.; Kozial, J.; Burstein, S.: Human recombinant erythropoietin promotes differentiation of murine megakaryocytes in vitro. J. clin. Invest *79:* 286–289 (1987).

Dr. R. Burghard, Zentrum für Kinderheilkunde der Philipps-Universität, Deutschhausstrasse 12, D-3550 Marburg (FRG)

Discussion

Schaefer (Würzburg): Do you have any idea why the mean corpuscular volume is increasing in your patient?

Burghard: It has been shown that the mean corpuscular volume is not increasing when patients are not iron overloaded before erythropoietin treatment, but it has also been reported from adults that MCV increases when there is a state of iron overloading. I suppose that this indicates a shift from iron into newly formed erythrocytes, but I have no real explanation.

Schaefer: Did you look for vitamin B_{12} or folic acid?

Burghard: Yes, before transplantation and before starting of EPO treatment and it was normal at that time.

Koch: As you are now able to correct the anemia of this patient, isn't he a case for nephrectomy?

Burghard: Because of severe hypertension?

Koch: Yes.

Burghard: Yes, this is a reason for doing that and we plan it before the next transplantation.

Winearls (London): I would like to make two comments about the MCV. We actually observed that in the iron-overloaded patients in our initial pilot study the MCV goes up and stays up at between 105 and 110 fl.

Burghard: After how many months?

Winearls: 6 months. It is coming down very slowly. A raised MCV was observed in iron-loaded dialysis patients in a cross-sectional examination of patients in a dialysis unit in England, where there had previously been a policy of giving the patients regular intravenous iron. There was quite a nice correlation between MCV and iron overload and the reason for this is not known. My second question is on a different subject. This sort of patient is a very obvious candidate for erythropoietin treatment. Can you just rehearse for us the arguments that removal of iron will actually reduce tissue injury in such patients. Does this occur, for example, in thalassemia? Do you expect the tissue damage in the heart and the liver to actually regress after iron removal and what is the evidence?

Burghard: In our patients there is no evidence so far. We did a liver scan before the institution of erythropoetin treatment and the density was increased. This child had cardiac dysrhythmias before EPO treatment requiring a pacemaker but sonography of the heart showed a normal ejection fraction and contractility before and after treatment. A second liver CT scan was not yet performed, and I think future investigations are required to answer your question definitively.

Winearls: I understand. I was hoping that the hematologists in the audience might be able to tell us whether there is evidence that iron removal in other situations, not in dialysis patients, makes any difference to tissue damage. Because otherwise – although it would be a good idea to give EPO treatment to free patients from the need for future transfusions – there is not actually a case for an aggressive policy of removing iron.

Bergström (Huddinge): Is there any hematologist here who would like to comment?

Caro: There are a couple of comments I would like to make. I think the increase in MCV is probably due to the high reticulocyte count. If you do not seem to observe it in other patients this could be because you do not have this excess of iron. The reticulocytes normally have the larger MCV. But if you do not have iron to fill them up with hemoglobin you may not see this increase of MCV. But it is a normal response if you have enough iron as, for example, in hemolytic anemias. The second thing I would like to mention is: You said you did liver scans. I do not know what you actually did. But the best way to follow iron overload, at least in the liver, and we are doing that routinely in patients with primary hemosiderosis, is using NMR studies of the liver. It gives a pretty good indication of the iron status of the liver. So I would recommend, in those patients, to do NMR studies before and after venesection.

Burghard: I agree with you. We first did computer tomography.

Caro: Coming back to your comment about the evidence for curing tissue damage by removal of excess iron: There is not that good evidence that once damage is established it can be improved. In the liver there is evidence that there may be some improvement. But in the heart there are very little data to suggest that once damage in the heart occurs that there is improvement following iron removal.

Müller-Wiefel: Are you sure that the very high dosage of captopril of 150 mg has not contributed a great deal to the reduced erythropoiesis in your child?

Burghard: I am not sure. But this antihypertensive treatment was the only way to cut the blood pressure peaks. This is an extremely high dosage of all antihypertensive drugs indeed.

Winearls: I cannot let Dr. Caro get away with the explanation of reticulocytosis being the cause for the high MCV. It is not related to the reticulocyte count. It would not explain why you get a high MCV in iron-loaded patients who are not on erythropoietin. One explanation is that this is a stress effect on the marrow that means that the red cells skip generations and so rather large red cells are produced. I should add, of course, that the vitamin B_{12} and folate levels were normal in these patients.

Eschbach: I think that we are observing two phenomena in the iron-overloaded patients to account for the increase in the MCV. Patients that are iron-overloaded have a high MCV, and superimposed on this baseline macrocytosis rhEPO treatment increases the MCV further because of a shift of the larger marrow reticulocytes out into circulation.

Müller-Wiefel: How long does it last?

Eschbach: It can last a long time!

Burghard: Up to the normalization of serum ferritin?

Eschbach: No iron-overloaded patient has yet had a normalization of his ferritin level. I would not expect the MCV to normalize until the iron overload condition resolves. On the other hand, I have cared for a hemodialysis patient who also has primary hemochromatosis and macrocytosis. Prior to dialysis, repetitive phlebotomy over several years reduced her serum ferritin level from 18,000 to 5,000 ng/ml. After 3–4 years of hemodialysis with its associated dialyzer blood loss, her ferritin level has been in the normal range for the past year. She continues to have a MCV of 110. The explanation for why iron-overloaded patients have a macrocytosis is not known to me, but it is not related to folic acid or B_{12} deficiency.

Caro: I would like to comment a little on this ferritin business. I would not expect the ferritin level to completely normalize because the amount of iron that you would be shifting from stores to red cells will depend on the amount of increase in hemoglobin and that is limited by how much you can improve it. You start with 7 g of hemoglobin, you go up to 12 g and then the iron stores will remain the same. So, if you start with a patient that has 10 g of iron overload and, in order to produce the additional red cells when you give erythropoietin, you use 3 g. The other 7 g of iron will remain there. They will not be excreted, unless you do venescetion or something else. I would not expect that the ferritin level will acutely reverse in these patients, unless you do something else. On the other hand there is a continuous blood loss due to the dialysis procedure, which in the long run will help to get rid of the excess of iron.

Burghard: I would agree with you that only erythropoetin and concomitant venesections may reduce the iron stores sufficiently.

Contr. Nephrol., vol. 66, pp. 149–155 (Karger, Basel 1988)

Urea Kinetics in Patients on Regular Dialysis Treatment before and after Treatment with Recombinant Human Erythropoietin

E. Zehnter[a], *M. Pollok*[a], *D. Ziegenhagen*[a], *P. Bramsiepe*[a], *F. Longere*[a], *C. A. Baldamus*[a], *U. Wellner*[b], *W. Waters*[b]

[a]Medical Clinic I, Department of Nephrology, and [b]Institute for Clinical and Experimental Nuclear Medicine, University Clinic, Cologne, FRG

Renal anemia is a regular finding in regular dialysis treatment (RDT) patients. Besides hemolysis, increased blood loss and toxic inhibition of hematopoiesis, the decreased erythropoietin (EPO) production is the main cause in the pathogenesis of renal anemia. Although EPO plasma concentration is increased in most RDT patients in spite of the loss of excretory renal function, the EPO concentration in relation to the degree of anemia is far too low [1–3, 11, 12, 15].

Since 1984, the molecular structure of human EPO is known and it is now produced by use of gene technology [4]. It became available for clinical trials in 1985 and the first clinical results in RDT patients were published late in 1986 [6, 12]. In 1987, further results were reported [5, 13, 14]. A dose-dependent increase in hemoglobin, and as the result of corrected anemia, an improved well-being and physical fitness of the patients were the clinically most evident findings [5, 6, 12, 13]. As side-effects, cardio-vascular complications and hypertension were noticed. Some investigators reported an increase in pretreatment urea and creatinine levels. This was either interpreted as an increase in protein intake or as a decrease in dialysis efficiency [5, 6, 14]. To answer the question whether the improved hematocrit and the EPO-induced increase in thrombocytes reduce dialysis efficiency or whether increased protein intake has an impact on protein metabolism, we applied urea kinetics to 10 RDT patients and measured body weight, total body potassium and pretreatment serum creatinine in relation to EPO-induced correction of renal anemia.

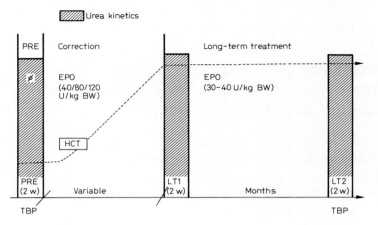

Fig. 1. Study design.

Patients and Methods

Patients. Ten stable anuric hemodialysis patients (6 male, 4 female), mean age 49.3 years (27–67), mean time on RDT 4.9 years (2–7), were included in the study. The underlying renal disease was glomerulonephritis in 4 patients, interstitial nephritis in 3, and unknown in 3. Hemodialysis treatment time was 4–5 h three times weekly according to individual needs. The individual dialysis schedule was kept constant during the study period. There were no dietary limitations with the exception of potassium restriction.

Measurements. Hematocrit (HCT) and serum creatinine were measured before dialysis (HD), and serum urea (U) and body weight (BW) before and after dialysis. Total body potassium (TBP) was determined by ^{40}K counting in a body counter [7] in 4 patients in the prephase and repeated in long-term phase 2 (LT2). As a parameter of dialysis efficiency the ratio of post- to predialysis serum urea levels were calculated (c_t/c_0). From the pre- and postdialysis serum urea concentrations, BW, and time intervals between consecutive HDs, urea generation rate (UGR) and protein catabolic rate (PCR) were calculated in the classical manner [8, 9].

Study Design. The time course of the study was divided into four parts (fig. 1). The prephase began 2 weeks before EPO application. The data were measured during every dialysis and mean values were calculated. During the correction phase, patients were treated with EPO given at the end of each dialysis. Four patients received 40 U/kg BW, 2 patients 80 U/kg BW, and 4 patients 120 U/kg BW until the HCT had risen for more than 10 vol% or until a HCT of 35 vol% was reached. In the then following long-term phase 1 (LT1) the dose was reduced to maintenance levels (30–40 U/kg BW, three times weekly). A repetitive measurement for a period of 2 weeks (LT2) was performed after 4 months at stable target HCT (fig. 1).

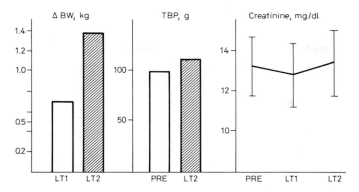

Fig. 2. Changes in BW, TBP and creatinine.

Table I. Results in urea kinetics (n = 10)

	HCT, %	Urea midweek pre-HD, mg/dl	UGR, mg/min	PCR, g/kg/day
PRE	22	146	15.4	1.2
LT1	32	149	16.0	1.2
LT2	29	126	13.6	1.2

Results

HCT increased in all patients from a mean value of 22% to 32% in LT1. The required time for this correction of anemia was EPO dose dependent. Midweek predialysis urea levels remained stable but showed a slight decrease in LT2. Dialysis efficiency was constant. Intratreatment symptomatology forced us to increase dry BW (post dialysis BW) in nearly all patients. The mean dry BW increased by 1.4 kg from PRE to LT2 (fig. 2).

Pretreatment serum creatinine levels remained unchanged. Mean TBP increased from 100.70 to 108.45 g, set in correlation to BW the ratio TBP/kg BW increased from 1.57 to 1.72. UGR increased slightly in LT1 but decreased to 13.57 mg/min in LT2. PCR remained constant (table I).

Discussion

As expected, HCT increased in all patients to the target value between 30 and 35 vol%. All patients felt better and reported an improved physical fitness and appetite. There were no changes in the dialysis regimen. Time on HD, blood flow and the dialyzer were kept constant. We found no increase in midweek predialysis levels of urea and creatinine. Dialysis efficiency characterized by c_t/c_0 remained constant throughout. This settles the question whether the increased HCT influences dialysis efficiency significantly. It must be pointed out, however, that heparin dosage was increased on an empirical basis from ca. 10,000 in PRE to ca. 15,000 U/HD in LT2. HCT-dependent deterioration of HD efficiency might become evident in short-hour high-efficiency HD [13].

Correction of anemia by EPO seems to have an anabolic effect indicated by a necessary increase of dry BW and by an increase in TBP. The question whether EPO directly causes this anabolism or whether it is the result of an increased physical fitness, indirectly caused by EPO-corrected anemia, remains unsettled. During the early correction phase when HCT was not yet increased, no changes in urea kinetics were noticed. Not even patients on the highest EPO dosage reported an increased food intake before HCT had risen.

The unexpected finding that UGR and PCR did not change during the entire study, in spite of the fact that TBP and dry BW increased, needs to be explained. If dialysis efficiency remained constant the reported improved appetite in a steady-state situation should result in an increased predialysis serum urea concentration as found by some investigators [14]. In our patients, midweek predialysis serum urea concentration remained unchanged throughout and so did UGR and PCR although patients reported an increased food and protein intake. The only explanation of this discrepancy is that patients were not in a steady state. In this new situation with increased food intake but constant UGR, the nitrogen balance can only be maintained by an increase in the body nitrogen inventory, that is lean body mass. Our parameters TBP and dry BW very strongly support this interpretation.

On the other hand, our study shows how misleading urea kinetics are if only UGR and PCR are taken as indicators for the nutritional status of patients. In any nonsteady-state situation – and this can be excluded – additional parameters like dietary protein intake or lean body mass are necessary. Only then are urea kinetics a meaningful parameter to follow the nutritional status of ESRD patients.

How reliable are parameters like increased dry BW and TBP as indicators for increased lean body mass? As pointed out in the Methods, dry BW had to be increased if hypotension and/or muscle cramps occurred regularly at the end of HD. Although it is a very subjective parameter, the fact that BW had to be increased in 7 of our 10 patients and that it was raised continuously up to a mean of 1.4 kg within 4 months is very suggestive that lean body mass had increased. Determination of TBP in a well-shielded body counter is a very reliable method with an error of $\pm 4\%$ [10, 16]. The mean change in our 4 patients is about 8% and therefore has to be interpreted as a real increase of body cell mass.

References

1   Caro, J.; Brown, S.; Miller, O.; Murray, T.; Erslev, A. J.: Erythropoietin levels in uremic nephric and anephric patients. J. Lab. clin. Med. 93: 449–458 (1979).
2   McGonigle, R. J. S.; Wallin, J. D.; Shadduck, R. K.; Fischer, J. W.: Erythropoietin deficiency and inhibition of erythropoiesis in renal insufficiency. Kidney int, 25: 437–444 (1984).
3   Radtke, H. W.; Claussner, A.; Erbes, P. M.; Scheuermann, E. H.; Schoeppe, W.; Koch, K. M.: Serum eryhtropoietin concentration in chronic renal failure: relationship to degree of anemia and excretory renal function. Blood 54: 877–884 (1979).
4   Lin, F. K.; Suggs, S.; Lin, C. H.; Browne, J. K.; Smalling, R.; Egrie, J. C.; Chen, K. K.; Fox, G. M.; Martin, F.; Stabinsky, Z.; Badrawi, S. M.; Lai, P. H.; Goldwasser, E.: Cloning and expression of the human erythropoietin gene. Proc. Natn. Acad. Sci. USA 82: 7580–7584 (1985).
5   Eschbach, J. W.; Egrie, J. C.; Downing, M. R.; Browne, J. K.; Adamson, J. W.: Correction of the anaemia of end-stage renal disease (ESRD) with recombinant human erythropoietin (rHuEPO): Results of a phase I–II clinical trial. Kidney int. 31: 198 (1987).
6   Winearls, C. G.; Oliver, D. O.; Pippard, M. J.; Reid, C.; Downing, M. R.; Cotes, P. M.: Effect of human erythropoietin derived from recombinant DNA on the anaemia of patients maintained by chronic hemodialysis. Lancet ii: 1175–1178 (1986).
7   Hughes, D.; Williams, R.: The calibration of a whole body radioactivity counter for the measurement of body potassium content in clinical studies. Clin. Sci. 32: 495–502 (1967).
8   Sargent, J. A.; Gotch, F. A.: Principles and biophysics of dialysis: in Drukker, Replacement of renal function by dialysis; 2nd ed., pp. 53–96 (Nijhoff, Dordrecht 1986).
9   Farrell, P. C.: Kinetic modeling in hemodialysis: in Nissenson, Fine, Gentile, Clinical dialysis, pp. 141–160 (Appleton-Century-Crofts, Norwalk 1984).
10 Pierson, R. N.; Wang, J.; Thornton, J. C.; Van Itallie, T. B.; Colt, E. W. D.: Body

potassium by four-pi ^{40}K counting: an anthropometric correction. Am. J. Physiol. *246:* F234–F239 (1984).

11   Summerfield, G. P.; Gyde, O. H. B.; Forbes, A. M. W.; Goldsmith, H. J.; Bellingham, A. J.: Haemoglobin concentration and serum erythropoietin in renal dialysis and transplant patients. Scand. J. Haematol. *30:* 389–400 (1983).

12   Zins, B.; Drüeke, T.; Zingraff, J.; Bererhi, L.; Kreis. H.; Naret, C.; Delons, S.; Castaigne, H. P.; Peterlongo, F.; Casadevall, N.: Erythropoietin treatment in anaemic patients on hemodialysis. Lancet *ii:* 1329 (1986).

13   Eschbach, J. W.; Egrie, J. C.; Downing, M. R.; Browne, J. K.; Adamson, J. W.: Correction of the anaemia of end-stage renal disease with recombinant human erythropoietin: Results of a phase I–II clinical trial. New Engl. J. Med. *316:* 73–78 (1987).

14   Editorial: Erythropoietin. Lancet *i:* 781–782 (1987).

15   Chandra, M.; Miller, M. E.; Garcia, J. F.; Mossey, R. T.; McVicar, M.: Serum immunoreactive erythropoietin levels in patients with polycystic kidney disease as compared with other hemodialysis patients. Nephron *39:* 26–29 (1985).

16   Morgan, D. B.; Burkinshaw, L.: Estimation of non-fat tissues from measurements of skinfold thickness, total body potassium and total body nitrogen. Clin. Sci. *65:* 407–414 (1983).

C. A. Baldamus, MD, Medizinische Universitätsklinik I,
Joseph-Stelzmann-Strasse 9, D-5000 Köln 41 (FRG)

Discussion

Eschbach: I want to comment on your results. It is the first time such a study has been done. We, too, have attempted to calculate the caloric intake of these patients and found it was very difficult. Although the patients describe how much more they are eating, it is difficult to document. Our dieticians have been very frustrated in trying to get good dietary intake records from the patients. So, I am interested in your and Dr. Bergström's comments on how to better analyze the food intake of these patients.

Baldamus: My comment to this is that usually you apply urea kinetics and assume the patients are in steady state. But these patients ar not in steady state. So, urea kinetics are really a misleading figure to use by themselves. For those of you who are planning to apply urea kinetics I just want to warn you in this regard.

Bergström (Huddinge): Well, I think that sooner or later these patients must be in steady state because they are not growing indefinitely. I would guess that at the time of your last measurements the urea generation rate would reflect how much protein they are eating. Don't you think so?

Baldamus: I agree absolutely. As soon as they are in steady state or have reached the new steady state at a higher protein intake level, urea generation certainly reflects protein intake. But as long as this steady state is not reached – and it is difficult to determine when it is reached – you are lost when you apply urea kinetics alone because dietary intake is impossible to estimate by dietary protocol. You need a second indicator for the body nitrogen inventory. We have to do this indirectly, I think, for instance, as in our case, by measuring total body potassium.

Winearls (London): I have two questions: If the mean body mass rises, some of this would be due to an increase in muscle mass. Would you not therefore expect the predialysis creatinine to rise?

Baldamus: Yes. But if you calculate the increase of muscle mass from the increase of total body potassium, this increase is small to show you a significant increase in creatinine. This issue, however, is the reason why I showed you how the predialysis creatinine behaved. So far, we could not find any significant change throughout.

Winearls: My second question is: You showed us the ratio between predialysis urea and postdialysis urea to look at dialysis efficiency. I am told that that is not a terribly accurate way of telling how efficient dialysis is. What you should do is to ensure that there is a steady TMP and the blood flows are exactly the same at the times of measurement. I wondered whether you made an attempt to measure creatinine clearance on the dialyser at two hematocrits, the low hematocrit and the high hematocrit.

Baldamus: No, I do not agree with you that creatinine is a more reliable parameter than urea for dialysis efficiency. Creatinine has a smaller mass transfer coefficient than urea and does not equilibrate instantaneously within the dialyzer. The same is true for any other intracellular solute which does not equilibrate instantaneously. Its clearance is no longer determined by the dialyzer but rather by the cell membrane. In my view urea is the most valuable parameter to calculate how efficient dialysis is.

Winearls: But if the plasma volume was changed there is less plasma going around the dialyzer and because you have a slow equilibration of creatinine you may expect the creatinine to behave differently from urea. Did you look at the ratio between predialysis and postdialysis creatinine in the same way that you looked at the predialysis and postdialysis urea.

Baldamus: We have not calculated that.

Bommer: Have you measured the muscle strength as another parameter of increased muscle mass in your patients, for example, by the handgrip test?

Baldamus: No we have not.

Wizemann (Giessen): You could not show a change in the ratio CT/CO and so there is no change in the KT/V. However, do you think the interaction of EPO might have an impact on the dialysis regimen? Especially when a very short duration of dialysis is being used?

Baldamus: We use a very conservative dialysis regimen of 4–6 h of dialysis. We end up with a urea clearance of about 150–160 ml/min, which is rather low. This facilitates equilibrium within the dialyzer, especially of substances which have not such a high transfer coefficient as urea has. One might run into real problems if one treats patients with very short high efficiency dialysis even when KT/V remains the same.

Contr. Nephrol., vol. 66, pp. 156–164 (Karger, Basel 1988)

Effect of Erythropoietin on Iron Kinetics in Patients with End-Stage Renal Disease

W. Waters[a], *U. Wellner*[a], *C. A. Baldamus*[b], *P. Bramsiepe*[b], *H. Schicha*[a, 1]

[a]Institut für klinische und experimentelle Nuklearmedizin der Universität und
[b]Medizinische Klinik I der Universität Köln, BRD

Most of the information about the different stages of erythropoietic cells and their control by erythropoietin (EPO) has been derived from in vitro studies. EPO is said to enhance the production of red cells mainly by amplifying the pool of erythrocytic progenitors [4]. As the description of EPO effects at the cellular level is not yet complete, a prediction on iron kinetics in the whole-body system remains speculative. Therefore, the aim of our study was to measure the EPO effect on iron kinetics using a complex model in patients with renal anemia on regular dialysis treatment.

Patients

Nine patients on regular dialysis treatment were investigated. The measurements were repeated in 4 of these patients when the stable target hematocrit had been established for 4 months. Four patients were measured during the correction phase of anemia. The EPO dosage of the long-term follow-up was 30–50 U/kg BW, during the correction phase three groups were formed, given either 40, 80 or 120 U/kg BW.

Methods

Iron Absorption
Radioiron retention was measured in a whole-body counter 20 min and 1 week after oral administration of 0.5 mg $FeSO_4 \cdot 7H_2O$ containing 0.5 µCi (19 kBq) ^{59}Fe.

[1] Thanks are due to G. Stanke and E. Seifert for expert technical assistance.

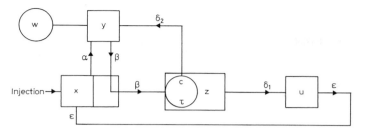

Fig. 1. Model of iron kinetics. Pools: x = quantity of iron essentially in plasma; y = labile iron pool; c = iron pool of the medullary region (bone marrow); z = erythrocytic iron pool; u = hemolytic iron pool; w = storage iron pool.

Iron Kinetics

^{59}Fe-labelled plasma (20 μCi; 740 kBq) and ^{51}Cr-labelled patient's erythrocytes (50 μCi; 1.8 MBq) were injected simultaneously. Radioactivity was measured at different organ sites using a probe detector over heart, spleen, liver and sacrum 10, 30, 60, 120, 180, 300 min and 1, 3, 6, 9 and 15 days after the injection. Blood samples were taken at the same time marks. The radioactivities of both radionuclides were measured in a gamma spectrometer. The ratio of measured blood radioactivity to the injected amount of radioactivity was calculated and is given as percentage for the different time marks. These date were further applied for the four-compartment model of iron kinetics (fig. 1) [6].

The model is based on the assumption that body iron mass is conserved throughout the time of measurement, i. e. 15 days. Marked iron losses or iron administration during this time affect the model and must be prevented. In normal men, 2 g of iron circulate in the red cells with a mean life span of about 120 days. The turnover of erythrocyte iron is therefore 17 mg/day. Blood volume and virtual life span of the erythrocytes are measured by means of ^{51}Cr-labelled erythrocytes.

The distribution of iron in the different compartments can be calculated from the disappearance of radioiron from the plasma and utilization curves (fig. 2). In coupled multicompartment systems the features of a single compartment cannot be obtained directly by the observation of this compartment alone. Observable is only the sum of changes in a single compartment which are influenced by all others. The tracer kinetics of the single compartments are described by the solutions of the differential equations. The features of the compartments have to be deducted from these solutions of the differential equations. The features of a metabolic system are the pools and turnovers of all compartments. The general mathematical solutions [7] and those of iron kinetics [6, 7] are described elsewhere.

Concerning iron metabolism, the turnover of the different pools are determined by more than one elimination pathway. For example, iron is eliminated from the labile pool (y) into the storage pool (w) and into the bone marrow (c); it is eliminated from the bone marrow (c) into the erythrocyte iron pool (z) and back into the labile iron pool (y), if ineffective erythropoiesis occurs (fig. 1).

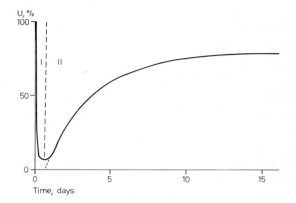

Fig. 2. Course of ^{59}Fe activity in the blood of a patient. I = ^{59}Fe disappearance from plasma; II = ^{59}Fe appearance in the erythrocytes – Fe utilization.

Results

From the probe measurements no overt extramedullary erythropoietic activity was detected in any patient. The following parameters showed no difference between the untreated and the EPO-treated groups: blood volume; plasma iron pool; exchangeable iron pool; hemolysis iron pool; erythroblast iron pool; marrow transit time of iron; iron absorption; erythrocyte iron utilization, and erythrocyte iron turnover.

Iron absorption was highly dependent on body iron stores, reflected by serum ferritin concentration. No effect of EPO treatment was detectable. Serum ferritin concentration and iron utilization were in good inverse correlation. EPO did not effect this.

The erythroblast iron pool was lower in untreated than in EPO-treated patients. It did not correlate with blood reticulocyte count. The half maximum time of the utilization curve reflects the output of erythrocytes from the bone marrow. The mean half maximum time is lower in the EPO-treated groups than in the untreated group. There seems to be a reduction of the variance in the treated groups, suggesting normalization (fig. 3).

As the half maximum time of utilization is dependent on the input function of iron into the bone marrow, we compared this parameter with the velocity of ^{59}Fe disappearance from the exchangeable iron pool (fig. 4). In those patients, in which the half-life of radioiron in the labile iron pool is higher than the half maximum time of utilization, high serum ferritin

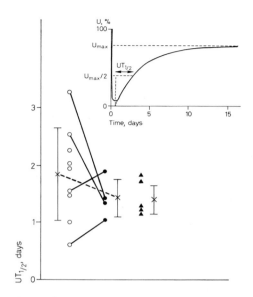

Fig. 3. Output velocity of erythrocytes from bone marrow, measured as the half maximum utilization time UT$_{1/2}$. o = Untreated; ▲ = EPO correction; ● = EPO long-term.

concentrations were found, suggesting a higher exchange of iron with the storage iron pool.

The output velocity of erythrocytes from the bone marrow, represented by the half maximum time of utilization, is in a narrower range in patients on EPO treatment and is independent from iron stores (fig. 5). The model allows to calculate the shunt iron turnover, indicating ineffective erythropoiesis. This is iron, which enters the bone marrow, but is not incorporated in circulating red cells. It reenters the exchangeable (labile) iron pool. It was calculated as percentage of the erythrocyte iron turnover.

Measuring the half-life time of ^{51}Cr-labelled erythrocytes and the ^{59}Fe erythrocyte turnover time, it was possible to calculate the life span of the red cells. In 3 patients with a short red cell life span this was drastically prolonged during EPO long-term treatment. On the other hand, in the 1 patient with a normal red cell life span it stayed normal. It needs to be stressed that in all 4 patients the hematocrit increased to the target value. The shunt iron turnover correlated well with the life span of erythrocytes. It is reduced under EPO long-term treatment in all 4 patients (fig. 6).

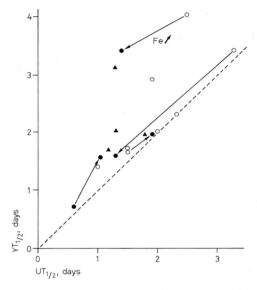

Fig. 4. Comparison of the half maximum utilization time with the half-life (YT$_{1/2}$) of ^{59}Fe in the labile (exchangeable) iron pool (y, see fig. 1). ○ = Untreated patients; ▲ = patients on EPO treatment during correction phase; ● = patients on long-term EPO treatment.

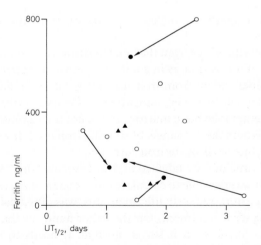

Fig. 5. Comparison of the half maximum utilization time (UT$_{1/2}$) with the serum ferritin concentration. ○ = Untreated patients; ▲ = patients on EPO treatment during correction phase; ▲ = patients on long-term EPO treatment.

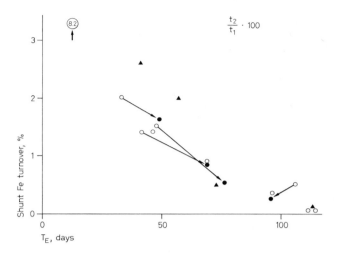

Fig. 6. Comparison of erythrocyte life span (T_E) with the bone marrow shunt iron turnover, which is given as percent of the erythrocyte iron turnover. t_2 = Shunt iron turnover; $t_2 = c \cdot \delta_2$, where c is bone marrow iron pool and δ_2 is elimination constant. t_1 = Erythrocyte iron turnover; $t_1 = z \cdot \delta_1$, where z is erythrocyte iron pool and δ_1 is elimination constant of erythrocyte degradation. (For symbols see also figure 1.) $\circ$ = Untreated patients; $\blacktriangle$ = patients on EPO treatment during correction phase; $\bullet$ = patients on long-term EPO treatment.

Discussion

Eschbach et al. [2] found in an uremic sheep model that by EPO treatment plasma iron turnover was elevated and the marrow transit time was shortened. This, however, was not found in our 4 reinvestigated patients under EPO treatment. The discrepancy can either be due to differences in methodology, to the small number of patients tested or to intermittent changes of iron stores. For longitudinal monitoring only model parameters which are independent from body iron stores, such as the life span of red cells, ineffective erythropoiesis (shunt iron turnover) and the output characteristics of labelled red cells from the bone marrow should be used.

From in vitro studies there exists some evidence on stimulating effects of EPO on identifiable precursor cells [3]. Bern and Goldwasser [1] found that 'marrow cells induced toward erythroid differentiation by treatment with erythropoietin respond by increasing the rates of iron uptake and hemoglobin synthesis'. The major effect at this stage of metabolism seems to be regulative in form of enhanced synthesis of porphobilinogen desaminase. The experiments suggest that the EPO response is due to transcription for porphobilinogen deaminase activity in form of de novo synthesis of this enyzme.

Other biochemical effects of EPO on the erythrocyte progenitor cells, such as the increase in RNA polymerase activity, nonhistone and histone protein synthesis, nuclear acetyl- and methyltransferase activity, DNA polymerase activity, DNA synthesis [5] and some other biochemical events, may be not only important for the enhancement of erythrocyte production, but also for the improvement of cell structures. This then may lead to an increased erythrocyte life span.

In 3 patients with an initially short red cell survival, EPO led to an enhancement of erythrocyte mass, which was due to enhanced production as well as to a concomitant prolongation of life span. In the 1 patient with a normal erythrocyte life span this was no further influenced by EPO. These data indicate that EPO improves not only the quantity of erythrocytes but also their quality restoring life span towards normal. The reduction of shunt iron turnover (ineffective erythropoiesis) by EPO treatment may be somehow involved in both effects.

References

1   Bern, N.; Goldwasser, E.: The regulation of bone biosynthesis during erythropoietin-induced erythroid differentiation. J. biol. Chem. *260:* 9251–9257 (1985).
2   Eschbach, J. W.; Mladenovic, J.; Garcia, J. F.; Wahl, P. W.; Adamson, J. W.: The anemia of chronic renal failure in sheep. J. clin. Invest. *74:* 434–441 (1984).
3   Goldwasser, E.: The action of erythropoietin as the inducer of erythroid differentiation. Hematopoietic stem cell physiology, pp. 77–84 (Liss, New York 1985).
4   Jelkmann, W.: Renal erythropoietin: Properties and production. Rev. Physiol. Biochem. Pharmacol. *104:* 139–215 (1986).
5   Spivak, J. L.: The mechanism of action of erythropoietin. Int. J. Cell Cloning *4:* 139–166 (1986).
6   Wellner, U.: Tracer in Lebewesen (Hippokrates, Stuttgart 1982).
7   Wellner, U.: Kinetic models of metabolism. Nucl. Med., Stuttgart *25:* 138–141 (1986).

Priv. Doz. Dr. med. Werner Waters, Institut für klinische und experimentelle Nuklearmedizin der Universität zu Köln, Joseph-Stelzmann-Strasse 9, D-5000 Köln 41 (FRG)

Discussion

Bommer: You measured the half maximum time of iron utilisation and you have correlated this value with ferritin. What is the correlation with the reticulocyte count in these patients? Have you correlated the iron utilisation rate with the reticulocyte count?

Waters: There was no correlation.

Bommer: I expect patients with a high reticulocytosis to have a high iron utilisation, a high iron incorporation into the reticulocytes and a high iron turnover. The utilisation rate is an index of iron utilisation, isn't it? So you must expect an increase if the reticulocyte count increases.

Waters: We expected it, really. But we did not find it. The explanation may be that the maturation of erythrocytes in the bone marrow is really affected by the EPO and maturation leads to stable precursor types of erythrocytes and the outlet from the bone marrow is, in some way, more effectively controlled.

Eschbach: I am not familiar with the model that you are using and I appreciated studying your paper. In contrast to your experience, we clearly showed a relationship between all the parameters that you mentioned. The reticulocytosis is correlated with both the plasma iron turnover which we have adjusted as the erythron transferrin uptake as well as with the marrow transit time. It correlates inversely with the marrow transit time and correlates positively with the red cell utilisation, at least in the 13 patients that we studied before and afterwards. I do not have a good explanation for why you did not show that correlation.

Waters: I think it is due to the changing situations in our patients. The situation before and after treatment in our patients was clearly not the same. Some of them got iron treatment. So far we cannot really compare, for example, mean plasma iron turnover as you did and we cannot compare the mean transit times. We can only say that in our patients before and after treatment we did not find statistically significant differences. I think we would have found them if the conditions were the same.

Eschbach: I recall that on one of your slides you showed the marrow transit time in 4 patients. Two showed a clear shortening in the marrow transit time as one would expect with rhEPO stimulation. The other 2 patients had baseline marrow transit times that were already very short, which doesn't make sense to me and implies that they were already being maximally stimulated with erythropoietin before they ever received exogenous EPO! So I am confused about your data.

Waters: It depends on the statistics and the comparable situations.

Winearls (London): Did I understand you correctly that you are finding a prolongation of the mean cell life span of the red cells after treatment as measured by the chromium technique.

Waters: Yes, there was a prolongation of virtual life span measured by chromium-labelled red cells. We corrected this life span by the iron turnover time. If the half-life of radiochromium-labelled erythrocytes is shortened you do not know whether it is due to hemolysis or to a shorter life span. Hemolysis was only slightly elevated and the reduction of life span seems to be really due to a shortened life span of the erythrocytes in patients without EPO treatment.

Winearls: Dr. Pippard has measured the red cell life span in our 10 patients. In 4 patients that we transfused there was an apparent increase in life span as you would expect because the measurement included transfused cells. There was no appreciable difference in the 6 untransfused patients. Were any of your patients transfused?

Waters: No, they were not.

Winearls: The second question is: Did you wait until the patients were in a steady state? At the second occasion that you measured the red cell life span, if you did not wait long enough, you would have a whole population of young cells which would appear to have a particularly long life span.

Waters: Yes, I think we measured after 4 months of long-term treatment and the mean life span was 50 days and the maximum 3 months. I think we waited about 2–3 life spans in the steady state before we started the second study.

Contr. Nephrol., vol. 66, pp. 165–175 (Karger, Basel 1988)

Effect of Erythropoietin Treatment on O$_2$ Affinity and Performance in Patients with Renal Anemia[1]

A. Böcker[a], *E. Reimers*[a], *B. Nonnast-Daniel*[a], *K. Kühn*[a],
K. M. Koch[a], *P. Scigalla*[b], *K.-M. Braumann*[a], *R. Brunkhorst*[a],
D. Böning[a]

[a] Abteilung für Sport- und Arbeitsphysiologie und Abteilung für Nephrologie der Medizinischen Hochschule Hannover, und [b] Boehringer Mannheim GmbH, Mannheim BRD

Compensation for the low oxygen capacity of blood in anemia takes place in different ways, e.g. by an increase of cardiac output and a right shift of the oxygen dissociation curve (ODC). The latter has the advantage to cost no extra energy. The O$_2$ extraction from blood during tissue passage is increased by a right-shifted ODC without decrease of capillary P$_{O_2}$ (fig. 1). As in many other types of anemia [2, 7], this mechanism is also reported in renal anemia [1, 12]. It is based on increased intraerythrocyte concentrations of organic phosphates, mainly 2,3-diphosphoglycerate (DPG), an intermediary product of glycolysis, which decreases hemoglobin-oxygen affinity. The aim of this study was to investigate changes of blood O$_2$ affinity and physical performance in renal anemic patients during treatment with recombinant human erythropoietin (rhEPO). One might expect that a marked decrease of the severity of anemia would result in normalization of O$_2$ affinity and DPG concentration.

Methods

Before and after treatment of 16 patients with renal anemia (4 females – mean age 51.7 years, 12 males – mean age 39.3 years, 3 smokers, 13 nonsmokers, not transfused, not nephrectomized, on regular hemodialysis) with rhEPO (Boehringer, Mannheim, FRG)

[1] Supported by Deutsche Forschungsgemeinschaft Bo360/5-1.

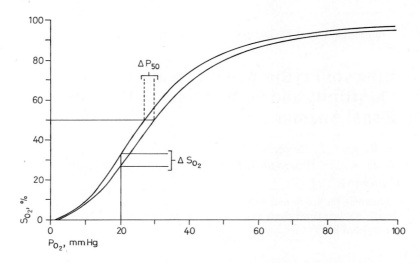

Fig. 1. Increase of O_2 extraction (Δ S_{O_2}) from blood with right-shifted ODC, latter quantified by the increase in P_{50} (Δ P_{50}).

40–120 U/kg, 3 times/week, for 50–101 days, mean 70.5 days, we determined 9.5–26 h after last dialysis the following:

(1) ODC at 6% CO_2 in the equilibration gases, with and without 10 mmol/l lactic acid, by use of Hemoxanalyzer (TCS, Southampton, USA) [5] connected to a BASIS 108 computer (BASIS Microcomputer GmbH, Münster, FRG) using own software for on-line data capture and data processing. Determination of standard half saturation pressure (P_{50}: P_{O_2} at 50% hemoglobin oxygen saturation, pH 7.4, temperature 37 °C, P_{CO_2} 42 mm Hg) as measure of oxygen affinity. Determination of Bohr coefficients (BC = δ log P_{O_2}/δpH) for correction of ODCs to various pH values.

(2) Hemoglobin (Hb), cyan-hemoglobin method, test kit (Merck, FRG).

(3) Hematocrit (Hct) value, microhematocrit centrifugation.

(4) DPG, enzymatically, test kit (Boehringer).

(5) Arterial pH (pH_a), in blood of the hyperemized earlobe, sampled in heparinized glass capillaries, with a blood gas analyzer BMS 2 (Radiometer, Copenhagen, Denmark). Correction to a Hct of 45% for the suspension effect on the liquid junction potential using the formula of Winslow et al. [15].

(6) Workload at a heart rate of 130 beats/min (PWC130), evaluated from a stepwise increasing bicycle ergometer test (25-W steps, 2 min each; ergometer: Jaeger, FRG). The heart rate was measured by ECG registration. All patients had been familiarized with the ergometric procedure. In 2 patients, who were exhausted with a heart rate lower than 130 beats/min, PWC 130 was determined by extrapolation. Data (P_{50}, DPG) of a group of 10 healthy male subjects served for comparison. The results of all measurements are presented as mean ± SD values. Statistical significance was determined by Student's t test.

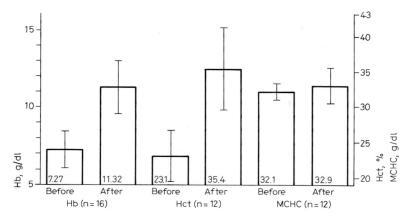

Fig. 2. Hb, Hct and MCHC before and after EPO treatment. Mean values in columns. Vertical bars represent SD.

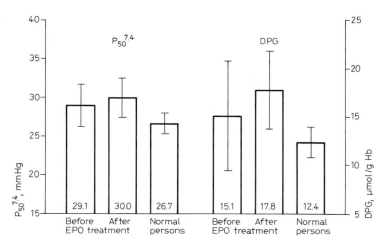

Fig. 3. P_{50} and DPG before and after EPO treatment compared to normal persons. Mean values in columns. Vertical bars represent represent SD.

Results

The most impressive result of EPO therapy was the significant (p<0.001) increase of Hb concentrations (from 7.3 ± 1.2 to 11.3 ± 1.7 g/dl, n=16) and Hct (from 23.1 ± 3.6 to $35.4 \pm 5.9\%$, n=12) (fig. 2). As expected in

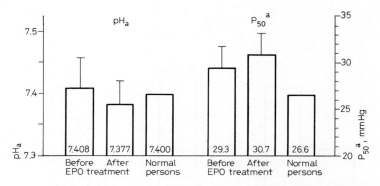

Fig. 4. Arterial pH and in vivo P_{50} in patients before and after EPO treatment compared to normal values. Mean values in columns. Vertical bars represent SD.

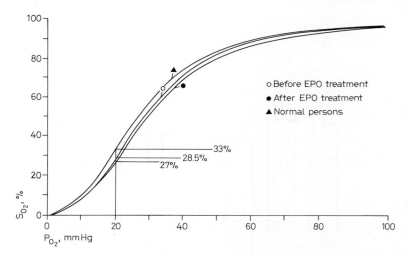

Fig. 5. Mean in vivo ODC of blood of patients before and after EPO treatment compared to normal persons.

renal anemia, MCHC was in a normal range (before treatment 32.1 ± 1.2 g/dl, after treatment 32.9 ± 2.4 g/dl, n=12) and did not change significantly. Prior to EPO therapy, mean standard P_{50} (fig. 3) was 29.1 ± 2.7 mm Hg (n=13). Although this is more than 2 mm Hg above that of the healthy persons (26.6 ± 1.2 mm Hg, n=10), the difference ist not signif-

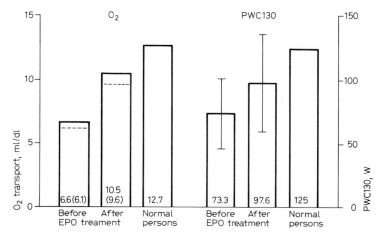

Fig. 6. Calculated O₂ transport and PWC130 in patients before and after EPO treatment compared to normal values. Mean values in columns. Vertical bars represent SD. Horizontal broken lines and values in parantheses represent O₂ transport without right shift of ODC.

icant because of a wide variation in the anemic patients. Likewise, DPG concentrations also varied considerably before treatment, with a mean of 15.2 ± 5.2 µmol/g Hb (n=16). Especially patients with relatively high Hb concentration had surprisingly low DPG concentrations. As in P_{50}, the difference to the group of healthy persons (12.4 ± 1.6 µmol/g Hb, n=10) is not significant. After EPO treatment, standard P_{50} was even higher (30.0 ± 2.6 mm Hg, n=16) in spite of markedly increased Hb concentration. The difference to the normal persons is now significant (p<0.01). DPG concentration (17.8 ± 4.1 µmol/g Hb) was significantly increased compared to pretreatment (15.2 ± 5.2 µmol/g Hb, p<0.02) as well as to normal subjects (12.4 ± 1.6 µmol/g Hb, p<0.001).

Arterial pH (Hct-corrected, fig. 4) in untreated patients was 7.408 ± 0.051 (n=13). After therapy it was decreased (not significantly) to 7.377 ± 0.038 (n=15). Calculation of the in vivo P_{50} (aP_{50}) via correction of P_{50} to pH$_a$ with individual Bohr coefficients resulted in 29.3 ± 2.3 mm Hg (n=10) before and 30.7 ± 2.4 mm Hg (n=15) after treatment (fig. 4). After therapy the mean in vivo ODC is more than 4 mm Hg right-shifted compared to normal persons (fig. 5).

The PWC130 (fig. 6) as a measure of aerobic performance was 73 ± 28 W (n=15) before and 98 ± 38 W (n=15) after treatment (compared to about 125 W in normal persons [11].) This increase is significant ($p < 0.05$). To exclude possible influences of application of β-blocking agents in 4 patients, we additionally tested the group without these persons. In this case the increase in PWC130 is even more impressive (74 ± 32 and 103 ± 39 W, $p < 0.01$).

Discussion

In general, blood of anemic patients has a lower O_2 affinity than that of normal subjects and correspondingly a right-shifted O_2 dissociation curve [2, 7, 13]. Investigations in persons with different types of anemia revealed mean standard P_{50}'s of more than 30 mm Hg [2, 7], P_{50} being negatively correlated to Hb concentration [6, 13]. For the mean Hb concentration of 7.27 g/dl before treatment, we expected a P_{50} of about 31 mm Hg when referring to these publications. The measured P_{50} of 29.1 mm Hg is, however, markedly lower. Such deviations in patients with renal anemia were found in several investigations.

In patients with a mean Hb of 6.9 g/dl (SEM ± 0.3), Humpeler et al. [7] obtained a standard P_{50} of 25.4 mm Hg (SEM ± 0.5), which was 1.8 mm Hg lower (!) than that of their normal persons. Mitchell and Pegrum [12] have reported a P_{50} of 29.3 mm Hg (SD ± 2.56) in a group of patients with a mean Hb of 6.0 g/dl. Blumberg [1] published a P_{50} of 27.9 mm Hg (SD ± 1.3) in renal anemia with a mean Hb concentration of 7.7 g/dl (SD ± 2.3). The P_{50} of his normal persons, however, was also very low (24.6 mm Hg). Assuming that this is due to the different method used in his investigation, the difference in P_{50} between healthy and anemic persons of about 3.3 mm Hg is similar to our findings. Finally, Lichtman [10] found 25.6 mm Hg immediately before dialysis.

Searching for reasons for the relatively high O_2 affinity in renal anemia we have to look for the main effector of Hb-oxygen affinity, DPG. Humpeler et al. [7] obtained 15.6 μmol/g Hb (SEM ± 0.9) and Lichtman [10] 15.6 μmol/g Hb (SEM ± 0.65), which are similar to our result of 15.2 μmol/g Hb before treatment. Blumberg [1] has communicated the DPG content per erythrocyte. Assuming a MCH of 30 pg, we calculate a DPG concentration of about 18 μmol/g Hb, which fits his higher difference between patients and normal persons in P_{50}. If compared to other types of anemia with similar Hb concentrations [2, 7], not only P_{50} but also in most cases DPG values of renal anemic patients are less. This is astonishing, since an additional factor possibly supporting DPG synthesis is the well-known hyperphosphatemia in these patients. This observation is in accordance with Lichtman and Miller [8].

Compared to normal persons, values for DPG (and therefore P_{50}) are extremely scattered. Causes of these differences among patients especially prior to therapy might be the large variation in blood pH and Hb concentration (quantified by the standard deviation). Alkalosis results in high, acidosis in low DPG-concentration, because of the pH optimum (pH 6.5) of the DPG decomposing enzyme 2,3-DPG phosphatase [4].

Hb increased markedly under EPO treatment. Knowing the negative correlation between Hb and P_{50}, we expected a decrease in P_{50} towards normal values, but the opposite happened: mean P_{50} increased slightly, thus becoming significantly different from the value of the normal persons. DPG concentration changed concomitantly. Interestingly these values are now in the range obtained in other types of anemia with similar Hb concentrations.

The behavior of DPG and P_{50} is unexpected for two reasons: Firstly, as mentioned above, the negative correlation of DPG and Hb [6] should lead to a decrease in DPG with increasing Hb. Secondly, while mean pH_a decreases, a lower DPG concentration would also be expected. There might be differences in erythrocyte constituents or in red cell environment causing the relatively low DPG concentration before treatment. Within the red cell, enzyme activity is important for metabolism. Young erythrocytes are known to possess high DPG levels resulting from high enzyme activities [14]. During the first time of EPO treatment the enhanced erythropoiesis leads to an increase of the young cells in erythrocyte population. However, the mean time of treatment between the two measurements was 70.5 days. Assuming that red cell survival time in renal anemia is shortened to about half that in normal persons [3], only in 6 patients with less than 60 days between the first and second test might a modest rejuvenation in mean cell age be present. There should be only a slight effect on the mean values of DPG and P_{50}.

A further factor possibly influencing blood O_2 affinity via DPG and ATP might be the extracellular concentration of inorganic phosphate. As known from routine examinations, there was an increase in plasma phosphate during treatment in most of the patients. Lichtman and Miller [8] found a significant correlation between ATP and phosphate, but there was no [9] or only a weak one [8] between DPG and phosphate. If there is an effect of inorganic phosphate on DPG concentration, it is certainly too small to reverse the influence of the Hb increase.

Thus it remains unclear, why P_{50} and DPG concentration are much lower than expected before treatment but correspond to Hb concentration after treatment. There are two possible explanations: (1) The age distribution of erythrocyte population is still not normal at the moment of the second measurement because of an increased lifespan of erythrocytes produced under EPO treatment. (2) Metabolism of erythrocytes produced before treatment is depressed (e.g. by a reduced enzyme equipment) and normalized in erythrocytes formed during treatment.

For estimation of the effect of the ODC right shift we assumed an arterial O_2 saturation of 96%, a constant pH and a tissue Po_2 of 20 mm Hg. Under these conditions, blood of healthy persons is desaturated in the capillary to about 33%, while O_2 saturation of patients' blood decreases to about 28.5% before and to 27% after treatment (fig. 5). Calculating the O_2 transport by 100 ml blood from lung to tissue, we obtained 6.6 ml O_2 before and 10.5 ml O_2 after treatment compared to about 12.7 ml O_2 in healthy subjects (fig. 6). The main reason for the increased O_2 transport is the rise in Hb concentration during treatment, but approximately 0.5 ml (7.5%) before and 0.9 ml (8.5%) after therapy are based on the right-shift of the ODC compared to healthy persons. As a consequence of these changes, tissue oxygen supply is possible with a lower heart rate than before treatment, which causes the significant increase of PWC130. The increase of PWC130 quantifies the considerable improvement of fitness and vitality noticed by the patients.

References

1 Blumberg, A.: Die renale Anämie (Huber, Bern 1972).

2 Böning, D.; Enciso, G.: Hemoglobin-oxygen affinity in anemia. Blut 54: 361–368 (1987).

3 Brenner, B. M.; Rector, F. C.: The kidney (Saunders, Philadelphia 1988).

4 Duhm, J.; Gerlach, E.: Metabolism and function of 2,3-diphosphoglycerate in red blood cells; in Greenwald, Jamieson, The human red cell, pp. 111–152 (Grune & Stratton, New York 1974).

5 Festa, R. S.; Asakura, T.: The use of an oxygen dissociation curve analyzer in transfusion therapy. Transfusion 19: 107–113 (1979).

6 Hjelm, M.: The content of 2,3-diphosphoglycerate and some other phosphocompounds in human erythrocytes from healthy adults and subjects with different types of anemia. Försvarsmedicin 5: 219–226 (1969).

7 Humpeler, E.; Amor, H.; Braunsteiner, H.: Unterschiedliche Sauerstoffaffinität des Hämoglobins bei Anämien verschiedener Ätiologie. Blut 29: 382–390 (1974).

8   Lichtman, M. A.; Miller, D. R.: Erythrocyte glycolysis, 2,3-diphosphoglycerate and adenosine triphosphate concentration in uremic subjects: Relationship to extracellular phosphate concentrations. J. Lab. clin. Med. *76:* 267–279 (1970).

9   Lichtman, M. A.; Murphy, M. S.; Byer, B. J.; Freeman, R. B.: Hemoglobin affinity for oxygen in chronic renal disease: The effect of hemodialysis. Blood *43:* 417–424 (1974).

10 Lichtman, M. A.: The effect of hemodialysis on the intraerythrocytic phosohate compounds and oxygen binding to hemoglobin. Kidney int. suppl. 2., pp. S134–S138 (1975).

11 Löllgen, H.: Kardiopulmonale Funktionsdiagnostik (Ciba-Geigy GmbH, Wehr/Baden 1983).

12 Mitchell, T. R.; Pegrum, G. D.: The oxygen affinity of hemoglobin in chronic renal failure. Br. J. Haemat. *21:* 463–472 (1971).

13 Rodman, T.; Close, H. P.; Purcell, M. K.: The oxyhemoglobin dissociation curve in anemia. Ann. intern. Med. *52:* 295–309 (1960).

14 Schmidt, W.; Böning, D.; Braumann, K.-M.: Red cell age effects on metabolism and oxygen affinity in humans. Resp. Physiol. *68:* 215–225 (1987).

15 Winslow, R. M.; Monge, C. C.; Staham, N. J.; Gibson, C. G.; Charache, S.; Whittembury, J.; Moran, O.; Berger, R. L: Variability of oxygen affinity of blood: Human subjects native to high altitude. J. appl. Physiol. *51:* 1411–1416 (1981).

A. Böcker, Abteilung Sport- und Arbeitsphysiologie, Medizinische Hochschule Hannover, Konstanty-Gutschow-Strasse 8, D-3000 Hannover 61 (FRG)

Discussion

Müller-Wiefel: Did you perform any studies of erythrocytes enzymes, for example of GOT?

Böcker: No.

Müller-Wiefel: You might have obtained information on the age of the erythrocyte population because the increase of 2,3-DPG would be the result of a younger and thus metabolically more active population of erythrocytes.

Böcker: That is a possible explanation. The problem is: The mean time between first and second investigation was 70 days. If the mean life span of erythrocytes – 60–80 days – did not change, there could have been only a slight effect of erythrocyte rejuvenation on the results, because only those persons treated for less than 60 days could have contributed. But the patients with a relatively short time, such as 50–60 days between the 1st and 2nd investigation, did not have extraordinarily high 2,3–DPG concentrations.

Eschbach: I missed the duration of the time between your studies. How long did they have a hematocrit of 35 before you repeated the studies?

Böcker: The mean time interval was 70 days between the 1st and 2nd investigations. There are some patients whose hematocrits were still increasing. But most were already in a stable state.

Eschbach: Why did you use a heart rate of 130? Is this your standard protocol or do you try to exercise your patients to exhaustion as we do?

Böcker: The problem is that they have a low physical performance, so we did it on a heart rate of 130 because at 150 or 170 we thought that we would have too many persons who do not reach this value.

Eschbach: That is what I think is interesting! We have been doing similar studies and have not found as good an improvement in exercise tolerance as you have. Your results are good, although your patients haven't improved back to normal. But, on the other hand, the hematocrit levels haven't been totally corrected yet either. So I am not sure what we can say except that they are getting better. We observed that patients 3 months after hematocrit stabilization aren't back to normal exercise tolerance and their heart rate fails to increase despite an increase in exercise ability. There is something that's keeping them from increasing their heart rate, even though they have a near normal hematocrit. I don't know whether this is from lack of conditioning or whether it is from chronic disease or both. This is an area that is going to need a lot of investigation but I think you have good preliminary data.

Böcker: In this respect I can say that we will have a third investigation. Maybe we will get more information at that time when the patients are in a steady state for a longer period of time.

Bauer: I think very important information for the clinician would be to have a simple test in order to assess physical performance and I just wonder what you would recommend to the clinician to assess physical fitness? We have heard a lot about this parameter and nobody has given any indication of what is actually meant with an increase in physical performance. I mean you should perhaps give some recommendations to those who would like to support their statements with facts.

Böcker: You mean information about the test we performed?

Bauer: That's right.

Böcker: It is a relatively simple test on a bicycle ergometer. However, you cannot take the patients without a pretest. They mostly do not know a bicycle ergometer and the whole machinery. After familiarization we test the patients on the ergometer by increasing the workload in steps of 25 W every 2 min up to a heart rate of 150. We did not want to exhaust them totally and did not reach heart rates higher than 150. The whole procedure takes no more than half an hour.

Böning: Of course it would be best to go to exhaustion. But we did not dare to do this with these patients. Therefore, we used the linear relation between load and heart rate. This is possible if you do not use beta-blocking agents which lower the heart rate. We did other measurements, for instance lactic acid from the ear lobe and pH. The results are not totally evaluated, but at least we know that the lactic acid concentration was lower at a given workload after hematocrits had increased. That is an additional parameter supplying information about the performance.

Wizemann (Giessen): You probably recorded the blood pressure during the exercise test. Was there any difference when patients had EPO or not?

Böcker: The evaluation of our data is not yet complete, so I cannot say anything about the behavior of blood pressure.

Bergström (Huddinge): I have a brief question to Dr. Eschbach: You mentioned that your patients failed to increase the heart rate when you exercised them. Is there any evidence that some of your patients might have autonomic neuropathy and that this could be the explanation?

Eschbach: I think that's theoretically a good explanation, except that clinically they did not have autonomic insufficiency. I'd like to support the concern of Dr. Bauer about standardization of exercise tolerance testing, but I also want to defend Dr. Böcker, who, I think, has a good testing method with the bicycle ergometer, which assesses oxygen utilization in these patients. But I do know that there are variations in how each center does the test. I hope the muscle physiologists standardize their tests so that we can compare tests from center to center.

Contr. Nephrol., vol. 66, pp. 176–184 (Karger, Basel 1988)

Correction of Renal Anaemia by Recombinant Human Erythropoietin: Effects on Myocardial Function

P. Grützmacher[a], *E. Scheuermann*[a], *I. Löw*[a], *M. Bergmann*[a], *K. Rauber*[b], *R. Baum*[c], *J. Heuser*[a], *W. Schoeppe*[a]

Departments of [a]Nephrology, [b]Radiology and [c]Nuclear Medicine, University Hospital, Frankfurt/M., FRG

In patients on maintenance haemodialysis, signs of impaired cardiac function and cardiomegaly are frequent. Many factors contribute to the pathogenesis including hypertension, fluid overload, arteriovenous fistula, electrolyte disorders, cardiac calcification, hormonal factors as hyperparathyroidism and catecholamine excess, carnitine deficit, toxic effects of uraemia on myocardial metabolism, pre-existing coronary and valvular heart disease and severe renal anaemia [Ikram et al., 1983; Drüeke and Le Pailleur, 1986]. In the present study, the effect of a correction of renal anaemia by recombinant human erythropoietin (rhEPO) on myocardial function was investigated.

Patients and Protocol

Eighteen patients on regular haemodialysis treatment (RDT) with severe renal anaemia but without need of blood transfusions during the last 6 months were treated with rhEPO (Boehringer Mannheim GmbH). According to a multicenter protocol, rhEPO was given intravenously three times weekly after haemodialysis using three different doses (40, 80 and 120 U/kg body weight) equally distributed among the group to increase the haematocrit from <28% either by 10 vol.% or to 35%. The dosis of rhEPO was then reduced to 10 U/kg and individually titrated to maintain the haematocrit between 30 and 35%.

One patient dropped out due to kidney transplantation. In the remaining 17 patients the mean haematocrit rose from 22.3% (19–26%) to 31.5% (30–33%). The investigations mentioned below were carried out in the anaemic state and when haematocrit values were stabilized at levels >30% for a mean of 12 weeks (5–19 weeks).

Hypertension was present in 10/17 patients prior to rhEPO therapy and in 11/17 patients after correction of anaemia. An increase of blood pressure was observed in 4 patients, 3 of these had preexisting hypertension, 1 normotensive patient became hypertensive under rhEPO therapy. In 2 hypertensive patients blood pressure decreased, 1 of these became completely normotensive requiring no further antihypertensive drugs.

Antihypertensive therapy consisted of converting enzyme inhibitors (n = 2), nifedipine (n = 6), verapamil (n = 2), other vasodilators (n = 3), β-blockers (n = 2) and nitrates (n = 3). Two patients were on digitoxin therapy because of a history of cardiac failure, although actually they were regarded as well compensated. As a worsening of hypertension was expected under rhEPO therapy [Winearls et al., 1986; Eschbach et al., 1987], and as a normal blood pressure profile has been achieved in all patients prior to rhEPO, the antihypertensive regimen was not changed to a uniform standard before rhEPO. However, it could be kept constant in most patients during the trial. Changes in this regimen included an increase or addition of nifedipine or nitrendipine (n = 3), an introduction of a combination of 50 mg dihydralazine and 240 mg verapamil (n = 1) as well as a reduction of captopril by 50% (n = 1) and an interruption of nifedipine (n = 1). Nifedipine was preferred because of its negligible negative inotropic and chronotropic effects. Mean body weight after haemodialysis did not change on rhEPO therapy; in each case, differences between dry body weight before and after correction of anaemia amounted to less than 0.5 kg.

Methods

A submaximal exercise electrocardiography (ECG) was carried out in 11 patients using a step-climbing test with identical loads before and after correction of anaemia. The loads were 50 W (n = 1), 75 W (n = 7), 100 W (n = 2) and 125 W (n = 1) over a period of 6 min. ECG was recorded at rest supine and upright, every minute during exercise and during a recovery period of a further 6 min. Heart rate was recorded continuously. Clinical symptoms, including dyspnoea, angina, sweating and exhaustion were registered by an uninformed technical assistant. Left ventricular hypertrophy, reflected by the (horizontal) Sokolow index (SV2 + RV5), and electrical myocardial axis reflected by the (frontal) angle α were calculated from an usual 12-lead ECG at supine rest in 17 patients. Upright posteroanterior and lateral chest X-rays were performed in 17 patients before and after correction of anaemia, always before haemodialysis. Cardiothoracic index, vascular pedicle width [Milne et al., 1984] and heart size were compared in a single blind fashion calculating an approximate heart volume using a standard formula [Frisch and Klepzig, 1983].

M-mode echocardiographic investigations were performed in 13 patients at rest. The following parameters were measured according to the guidelines of the American Society of Echocardiography [Sahn et al., 1987; Feigenbaum, 1985]: left ventricular end-diastolic and end-systolic diameter (LVED, LVSD), left ventricular end-diastolic and end-systolic volume (LVEDV, LVESV), thickness of the septum interventriculare (IVS) and the left ventricular posterior wall (LVPW).

Myocardial contractility at rest and during exercise was investigated in 9 patients, using fully automated sectorial equilibrium radionuclide ventriculography [Standtke et al., 1983]. Global EF and peak ejection rate (PER) were compared before and after correction of anaemia.

For statistical analysis Student's paired t-test was applied. Statistically significant differences were defined by a p value of less than 0.05.

Table I. Correction of renal anaemia by rhEPO in RDT patients (n = 11): effect on subjective exercise tolerance (step-climbing test)

Symptoms	Before	After
Dyspnoea	4	2
Angina	2	0
Exhaustion	7	4
Sweating	1	0.
Interruption	3	0

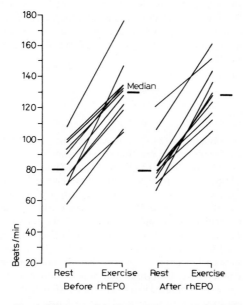

Fig. 1. Changes of the heart rate at rest and under submaximal physical exercise. The increase of heart rate under exercise was the same before and after correction of anaemia by rhEPO.

Results

Under exercise, a significant ST segment depression >0.2 mV occurred in 2 patients, which disappeared after correction of anaemia. Arrhythmias could not be observed in any patient. Limitation of physical working capacity led to the interruption of the exercise investigation in 3 patients

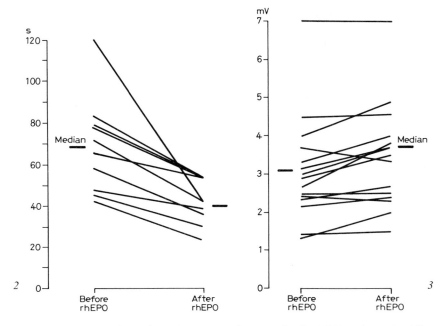

Fig. 2. Recovery time of the heart rate after exercise in RDT patients (n=10), expressed as the time (in seconds) until rate has recovered by 50% of the increase (t/2).

Fig. 3. Changes of Sokolow index after correction of anaemia by rhEPO in RDT patients.

before rhEPO. After correction of anaemia every patient tolerated the selected load. Exercise tolerance reflected by clinical symptoms markedly improved after correction of anaemia (table I).

The mean heart rate at rest as well as the absolute and relative increase under exercise were identical before and after correction of anaemia (fig. 1). However, the recovery time of the heart rate after exercise, expressed as t/2, was significantly lower ($p < 0.05$) in each case (fig. 2).

The Sokolow index calculated from ECG at rest exceeded the normal limit of 3.5 mV in 4 patients. After rhEPO therapy the median Sokolow index increased significantly ($p < 0.05$) from 3.2 mV (1.4–7.0 mV) to 3.7 mV (1.5–7.0 mV) (fig. 3), whereas the angle α remained constant at 28° (−2 to +57°) versus 29° (−3 to +53°).

Cardiothoracic index and vascular pedicle width on the upright PA chest X-ray did not change. However, the cardiac volume, calculable in 12 of

Table II. Correction of anaemia of RDT patients: effect on chest X-ray findings

Patient	Cardiothoracic index		Vascular pedicle width, mm		Heart volume, ml	
	before	after	before	after	before	after
1	0.49	0.47	50	49	750	710
2	0.41	0.43	54	51	–	810
3	0.52	0.52	66	72	740	630
4	0.51	0.53	50	53	870	800
5	0.62	0.63	52	56	830	990
6	0.51	0.46	63	58	970	800
7	0.45	0.43	54	51	580	580
8	0.51	0.51	76	70	920	860
9	0.49	0.51	69	70	–	–
10	0.67	0.65	59	51	590	610
11	0.54	0.55	56	62	–	730
12	0.45	0.43	55	55	590	580
13	0.50	0.52	65	68	990	1,110
Median	0.51	0.51	56	56	750	730

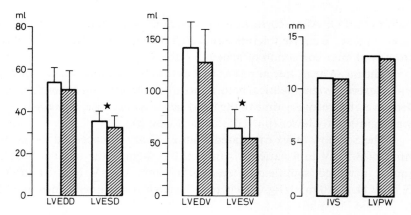

Fig. 4. Echocardiographic changes after correction of anaemia by rhEPO in RDT patients (n=13). Means ± SEM. □ = Before rhEPO, ▨ = after rhEPO. *p <0.05.

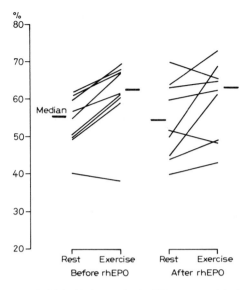

%

Fig. 5. Global left ventricular EF at rest and during exercise measured by equilibrium radionuclide ventriculography.

the 17 patients from cardiac diameters, decreased in 5 patients by $>5\%$, increased in 2 and remained constant ($\pm <5\%$) in the remaining 5 patients (table II).

Echocardiographic investigation of 13 patients disclosed a reduction of the mean LVEDD and LVESD as well as LVEDV and LVESV. Regarding LVESD and LVESV this reduction was significant. Thickness of the IVS and LVPW did not decrease (fig. 4).

Global left ventricular EF, measured by radionuclide ventriculography in 9 patients, was normal, i. e. $>50\%$, at rest in 8 patients and slightly decreased in 1 patient prior to EPO treatment. Under exercise all 8 showed a normal increase of EF. After correction of anemia no significant changes were observed (fig. 5). PER at rest and during exercise was not influenced by rhEPO therapy either.

Discussion

Data indicate a marked improvement of exercise tolerance by rhEPO therapy in the 2 patients with symptomatic coronary heart disease as well as in the other patients reflected by the relief of symptoms. Maximal physical working capacity was not measured in general, but improved in 3 patients submitted to a too high work load. Although the relative and absolute increase in heart rate under exercise was nearly unchanged, the recovery time of the heart rate after exercise was significantly lower after correction of anaemia. These findings suggest that renal anaemia contributes to a great extent to the reduced physical activity and exercise tolerance of many patients on RDT [Kettner et al., 1984].

Furthermore, correction of anaemia induced a measurable decrease in cardiac volume on chest X-ray controls. Correspondingly, a significant decrease in left ventricular volume could be detected by echocardiography. As prior to treatment nearly all patients presented with a normal heart size as determined by X-ray, these changes seem to indicate that renal anaemia induces a minor myocardial dilatation even in asymptomatic patients in whom anaemia was regarded 'as well compensated'. It seems noteworthy that the only increases in heart size as determined by X-ray were observed in patients with worsening of hypertension.

Although there were no changes in mean body weight after haemodialysis under rhEPO therapy and measurements were performed at comparable intervals to haemodialysis sessions in most cases, a possible influence of an inapparent relative increase in dry body weight cannot be completely excluded. On the other hand, there was no evidence for this assumption as judged from the patients' tolerance to volume reduction during dialysis.

Global left ventricular ejection fraction, already normal in most patients prior to treatment, was not influenced by correction of anaemia. The results of radionuclide ventriculography were confirmed by echocardiographic findings. Both methods usually show a good correlation [Reifart et al., 1984].

The small but significant increase of the Sokolow index, usually interpreted as an increase in left ventricular hypertrophy [Sokolow and McIllroy, 1979], is surprising. An increase of left ventricular hypertrophy could be due to an increase of myocardial afterload in case of worsening of hypertension. Actually mean blood pressure increased moderately in 4 patients within the normal range despite enhanced antihypertensive medication. Furthermore, functional myocardial characteristics could be influenced by a higher blood viscosity per se, also in the absence of a blood pressure increase, according to the rule of Hagen-Pouisseulle. However, echocardiographic measurements of the thickness of the septum interventriculare and left ventricular posterior wall rendered no evidence for an increased myocardial hypertrophy.

The interpretation of the increased Sokolow index as an improved electro-physical activity after correction of renal anemia remains speculative. Further studies, especially including patients with severe cardiac dysfunction, will probably provide more insight into the different effects of correction of anaemia on the uraemic myocardium.

References

Drüeke, T.; Le Pailleur, C.; Cardiomyopathy in patients on maintenance haemodialysis. Contr. Nephrol., vol. 52, pp. 27–33 (Karger, Basel 1986).

Eschbach, J. W.; Egrie, J. C.; Downing, M. R.; Brown, J. K.; Adamson, J. W.: Correction of the anemia of end-stage renal disease with recombinant human erythropoietin. New Engl. J. Med. *316:* 73–78 (1987).

Feigenbaum, H.: Echokardiographie, 2. Aufl. (Perimed, Erlangen 1985).

Frisch, P.; Klepzig, H.: Bedeutung und Durchführung von Herzvolumenbestimmungen, in Kaltenbach, Klepzig, Röntgenologische Herzvolumenbestimmung, pp. 1–9 (Springer, Berlin 1983).

Ikram, H.; Lynn, K. L.; Baylex, R. R.; Little, P. J.: Cardiovascular changes in chronic hemodialysis patients. Kidney int. *24:* 371–376 (1983).

Kettner, A.; Goldberg, A.; Hagberg, J.; Delmez, J.; Harter, H.: Cardiovascular and metabolic responses to submaximal exercise in hemodialysis patients. Kidney int. *26:* 66–71 (1984).

Milne, E. N. C.; Istolesi, M.; Miniati, M.; Giuntini, C.: The vascular pedicle of the heart and the vena azygos. Radiology *151:* 1–8 (1984).

Reifart, N.; Maul, F. D.; Mützel, E.; Sarai, K.; Hör, G.; Kaltenbach, M.; Satter, P.: Aortokoronare Bypass-Operation bei erheblich reduzierter linksventrikulärer Funktion infolge chronischer Ischämie. Dt. med. Wschr. *109:* 1671–1677 (1984).

Sahn, D. J.; DeMaria, A.; Kissko, J.; Weyman, A.: The Committee on M-mode standardization of the American Society of Echocardiography. Recommendations regarding quantitation in M-mode echocardiography: results of a survey of echocardiographic measurements. Circulation *58:* 1072–1083 (1978).

Sokolow, M.; McIllroy, M. B.: Clinical cardiology; 2nd ed. (Lange, Los Altos 1979).

Standtke, R.; Hör, G.; Maul, F.-D.: Fully automated sectorial equilibrium radionuclide ventriculography. Proposal of a method for routine use: exercise and follow-up. Eur. J. nucl. Med. *8:* 77-83 (1983).

Winearls, C. G.; Oliver, D. O.; Pippard, M. J.; Reid, C.; Downing, M. R.; Cotes, P. M.: Effect of human erythropoietin derived from recombinant DNA on the anaemia of patients maintained by chronic haemodialysis. Lancet *ii:* 1175–1178 (1986).

P. Grützmacher, MD, Department of Nephrology, Division of Internal Medicine, University Hospital, Theodor-Stern-Kai 7, D-6000 Frankfurt/Main (FRG)

Discussion

Wizemann (Giessen): Thank you for those beautiful results. We can confirm your impression that the ECG is not a good method to look for left ventricular hypertrophy. What I want to ask you is: you have measured just before and just after reaching the target of your EPO study. I think one has to follow up those patients to look at the development of left ventricular hypertrophy! One should expect that changes will come later. I hope we are able to demonstrate regression of hypertrophy measured by echocardiography.

Grützmacher: We should wait a little longer.

Winearls (London): Can I just ask when you did your chest X-rays and whether you made certain that you took them at exactly the same time in relation to dialysis?

Grützmacher: Yes. In the majority of the cases. The relation to dialysis was the same in nearly all the cases.

Winearls: Was it before dialysis?

Grützmacher: Always before dialysis. In some exceptional cases it was done the day after, but then the control was also made the day after. The changes in body weight during all these investigations were in every case actually less than 0.5 kg.

Bauer: Did you have a chance to calculate the peripheral resistance in the study?

Grützmacher: No, unfortunately not.

Bauer: But I think this can be done rather easily and it is very important to have this figure.

Grützmacher: We measured the cardiac output by echocardiography, but that is a very arbitrary method.

Bauer: I still think to calculate peripheral resistance is very easy even with such a method.

Grützmacher: I would like to do that using a better method to measure input parameters.

Wizemann: The increase in the ejection fraction following exercise demonstrates that you have researched a very healthy group of patients. Are you aware of, or is there anybody here who has experience with, treating patients with coronary artery disease? That would be a relevant population to study.

Grützmacher: Yes, that is a limitation of the study. We mostly included uncomplicated patients because, according to the protocol, we were obliged to take patients who tolerate anemia without transfusions. These are regularly patients with well-functioning heart.

Bahlmann: I would like to ask you how reliable are actually your cardiac output values? Because, on theoretical grounds, it is to be expected, also taking into account the results of animal experiments, that the cardiac output falls after correcting anemia.

Grützmacher: Yes, I agree completely. Calculating cardiac output by echocardiography means calculating a simple product of the stroke volume × pulse rate. According to echo specialists, it is a very crude method permitting only an estimate. I think this parameter is not reliable enough.

Bahlmann: And for that reason you cannot apply the equation for calculating total peripheral vascular resistance because you will not get any reliable result?

Grützmacher: Yes. That is why I have not done this.

Contr. Nephrol., vol. 66, pp. 185–194 (Karger, Basel 1988)

Effect of Treatment with Recombinant Human Erythropoietin on Peripheral Hemodynamics and Oxygenation

B. Nonnast-Daniel, A. Creutzig, K. Kühn, J. Bahlmann, E. Reimers, R. Brunkhorst, L. Caspary, K. M. Koch

Department Innere Medizin und Dermatologie, Abteilung Nephrologie und Abteilung Angiologie, Medizinische Hochschule Hannover, FRG

Chronic anemia in patients with end-stage renal disease (ESRD) is known to be associated with an increased cardiac output and a normal or a moderately lowered peripheral vascular resistance securing a sufficient oxygen supply to the peripheral tissues in spite of a reduced number of erythrocytes [6, 12, 15]. This constellation of central and peripheral hemodynamics was postulated to contribute to the development of hypertension in uremic patients [6, 15]. On the other hand, acute elevation of the hematocrit by transfusion in patients with ESRD is followed by a decrease of cardiac output and an increase of total peripheral vascular resistance resulting in an increase of diastolic blood pressure [15].

Since one major clinical complication of a therapy with recombinant human erythropoietin (rhEPO) in dialyzed patients may be the development of severe hypertension [11, 20], the following study was designed to further clarify the interrelation between peripheral vascular resistance, tissue oxygenation and blood pressure in chronic hemodialysis patients before and during a slow improvement of the hematocrit by rhEPO treatment. Hence calf blood flow, calculated peripheral vascular resistance and transcutaneous oxygen pressure as well as clinical parameters such as blood pressure, heart rate, X-ray cardiac diameter and hematocrit were investigated in 7 hemodialyzed patients before and after 3 months of rhEPO therapy.

Patients and Methods

Patients. Initially the study population consisted of 12 patients. All patients were severely anemic and participated in a multicenter trial of rhEPO in the treatment of anemia in ESRD. Five patients were on mild antihypertensive therapy with β-blockers and/or ACE inhibitors at the beginning of the study. In all of them the dose of antihypertensive drugs had to be increased in the course of rhEPO treatment. Because of the possible modifying influence of these drugs on hemodynamics, these 5 patients were excluded. The remaining 7 patients (2 women and 5 men; aged 22–57) were normotensive initially and remained so throughout the study without any antihypertensive medication; hemodialysis had been initiated due to chronic glomerulonephritis (n=3), chronic interstitial nephritis (n=3) and primary malignant hypertension (n=1).

Study Protocol. Measurements were performed 1 week before and 10–12 weeks after initiation of rhEPO. The patients received rhEPO intravenously three times weekly after dialysis in a randomized fashion: either 40 (n=2), 80 (n=3) or 120 (n=2) U rhEPO/kg.

Parameters Investigated. Heart rate was measured continuously by Holter monitoring over 30 min at the beginning of three consecutive dialyses and averaged. All other parameters were determined 12–20 h after dialysis. Blood pressure was measured by the cuff method on the arm and mean blood pressure was calculated as MAP = diastolic blood pressure $+\frac{1}{3}$ (systolic – diastolic blood pressure). Calf blood flow was measured using the venous occlusion plethysmography after a resting period of 30 min and expressed in ml/min/100 ml tissue [3, 4, 13, 17]. Blood flow was determined at both legs and averaged. Peripheral vascular resistance was calculated as MAP/blood flow (mm Hg/ml/min/100 ml). Transcutaneous O_2 pressure was measured using tcp-O_2 electrodes (TCMR, Radiometer, Copenhagen, Denmark) at 37 and 44 °C [7] electrode core temperature. In our laboratoy the normal values of healthy volunteers were 6.5 ±2.5 SD at 37 °C and 55 ±23 SD at 44 °C (n=10). In addition, hemoglobin (Hb) and hematocrit (Hct) were determined and the cardiac transversal diameter was measured with the help of chest X-ray.

Statistical evaluation was performed with the paired t-test; $p < 0.05$ was considered as indicator of significance.

Results

The mean values ± SD of the various parameters before and after correction of anemia by rhEPO treatment are listed in table I and in part are shown graphically in figure 1. Hematocrit increased significantly within the observation period from 21 to 33%. At the same time the mean heart rate and the cardiac transversal diameter decreased significantly. Patients were normotensive before rhEPO therapy, under rhEPO the systolic and diastolic blood pressure tended to rise but the increase was not significant whereas the calculated mean arterial blood pressure increased significantly. No antihy-

Table I. Hemodynamic studies in 7 uremic patients: mean values ± SD before (pre-EPO) and 10–12 weeks after start of rhEPO (EPO)

	MAP mm Hg	HR bpm	CTD cm	CBF ml/min/ 100 ml	PVR mm Hg/ ml/min/ 100 ml	tcp-O_2 44 °C torr	tcp-O_2 37 °C torr	Hct %	Hb g/dl
Pre-EPO	89.9 ± 10.7	77.9 ± 10.8	14.4 ± 1.5	4.5 ± 0.5	17.3 ± 1.5	31.5 ± 15.9	4.3 ± 3.7	20.7 ± 2.9	6.8 ± 1.0
	*	**	*	*	*	**	**	**	**
EPO	95.4 ± 12.3	68.3 ± 9.1	13.8 ± 1.6	3.1 ± 1.1	31.0 ± 13.1	43.7 ± 9.3	8.5 ± 6.4	33.1 ± 3.6	10.9 ± 1.2

MAP = Mean arterial blood pressure; HR = heart rate; CTD = cardiac transversal diameter; CBF = calf blood flow; PVR = peripheral vascular resistance; tcp-O_2 44 °C and tcp-O_2 37 °C = transcutaneous oxygen pressure. * p < 0.05; ** p < 0.001.

pertensive drug therapy had to be initiated. 'Dry' weight after dialysis did not change. The resting calf blood flow was in the upper normal range [3] and decreased significantly after rhEPO, but remained in the normal range. Accordingly the calculated regional vascular resistance was normal before rhEPO and rose significantly under rhEPO. Prior to rhEPO therapy the transcutaneous oxygen pressure of the forefoot was in the lower normal range. It rose significantly under rhEPO without exceeding the normal range. These results were found at 37 °C as well as at 44 °C electrode core temperature.

Discussion

The present study describes the hemodynamic response to a slow partial correction of renal anemia without clinically apparent accompanying changes of the volume status. In the normotensive patients the blood pressure rises significantly but does not reach hypertensive levels. The regional blood flow falls slightly but significantly. These changes reflect a significant increase of regional peripheral vascular resistance after 10–12 weeks of rhEPO treatment.

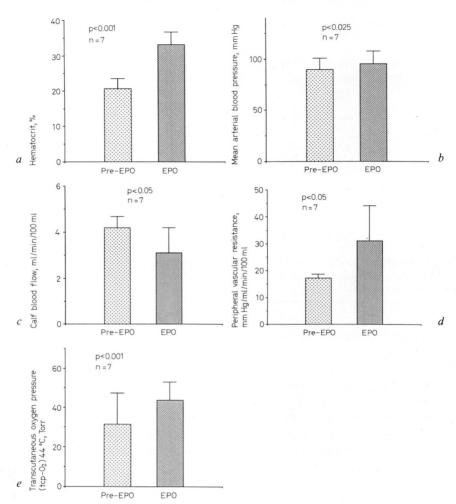

Fig. 1. Mean values ± SD of hematocrit *(a)*, MAP *(b)*, calf blood flow *(c)*, peripheral vascular resistance *(d)*, and transcutaneous oxygen pressure (at 44 °C) *(e)* before (pre-EPO) and 10–12 weeks after the start of rhEPO treatment (EPO).

Our results are similar to the effects of raising the hematocrit of uremic patients to normal by serial transfusions of packed red cells as described by Neff et al. [15]. These authors observed a rise in total peripheral vascular resistance together with a fall in cardiac output and a rise in blood pressure parallel to the increase in hematocrit. These alterations were induced by a relatively fast correction of anemia up to normal hematocrit values and they were reversible when anemia returned after stopping the transfusions. The significant slowing of the heart rate observed by us when anemia was corrected can be taken as an indicator of a decreased cardiac output. The heart rate was not only slower during rest but also during the stress of starting the dialysis procedure. The previous therapeutic trials with rhEPO reported an increase of blood pressure and even the development or worsening of hypertension [11, 20]. In principle our findings were similar. We not only observed an increase of mean arterial blood pressure in normotensives but also in the initially hypertensive patients the blood pressure could only be kept constant by increasing the dose of β-blockers. In another study with administration of rhEPO up to 40 weeks in dialysis patients it was also necessary to reinforce the antihypertensive therapy in patients already under antihypertensive treatment at the start of the study. Contrary to our results, no elevation of blood pressure was seen in normotensive patients [5].

Two mechanisms might be responsible for the rise in blood pressure during rhEPO treatment and correction of anemia: (1) higher blood viscosity due to a rise of total red cell mass causes an increase of total peripheral resistance, and (2) improvement of tissue oxygenation due to higher oxygen transport capacity increases arteriolar vascular tone and thereby total peripheral resistance. It was shown experimentally that hypoxia leads to a vasodilatation which is reversible after restoring normal oxygen supply [9, 10]. It is assumed that the vascular diameter is regulated locally by chemical vasoactive mediators [8, 10]. Because of the reduced oxygen transport capacity such mediators would accumulate in renal anemia and cause an autoregulatory vasodilatation which restores oxygen supply at least partially. Accordingly the increasing hematocrit during rhEPO therapy would lead to a better oxygen delivery and thereby to a reduction of vasodilatory mediators and a decrease of blood flow. To evaluate this concept more closely we measured the transcutaneous oxygen pressure of the forefoot at 37 °C and 44 °C, the latter state representing hyperemia. At 37 °C, transcutaneous oxygen pressure before rhEPO therapy was in the lower normal range. Since the transcutaneous oxygen pressure increased, the peripheral oxygen delivery obviously improved after raising the hematocrit. Thus the higher oxygen transport capacity due to increased red cell mass was not offset by a reduced blood flow. During local hyperemia at 44 °C the influence of local vasoconstriction is abolished and maximal transcutaneous oxygen tension is obtained. As was to be expected, a clear-cut significant increase of the transcutaneous oxygen pressure was found parallel to the higher hematocrit as a consequence of the higher oxygen transport capacity.

When transcutaneous oxygen pressure before rhEPO therapy is still within the normal range in spite of severe anemia, this is not only due to the reduced peripheral vascular tone and the rise in blood flow but also to the reduced hemoglobin oxygen affinity of patients with renal anemia [1, 14]. This latter mechanism was shown to be still operative after slow partial correction of renal anemia 12 weeks after the start of rhEPO treatment [2].

Changes of hematocrit itself have a known influence on microcirculation. The whole blood viscosity depends on hematocrit but the relation is not linear [16, 18, 19]. The increase in viscosity with rising hematocrit is less within the anemic range of hematocrit. This especially applies for hematocrits below 30% [19]. Furthermore, the influence of hematocrit on blood viscosity is dependent upon blood flow velocity and shear rate [18]. The effect of hematocrit on viscosity is less with higher blood flow velocity and shear rate. On the other hand, the influence of shear rate itself on viscosity is dependent on hematocrit and is smaller in anemia [18].

For this reason it is nearly impossible to estimate the influence of the various factors on blood flow viscosity when raising the hematocrit from 21 to 33% as in this study. The increase in blood viscosity certainly contributes to the observed increase of peripheral vascular resistance but the extent of this effect may be limited.

Summary and Conclusions

Slow progressive improvement of renal anemia from 21 up to 33% hematocrit by rhEPO treatment results in an increase of tissue oxygenation as indicated by a rise of the transcutaneous oxygen pressure. In normotensive patients this was accompanied by an increase in MAP (Δ 6 mm Hg) within the normal range and a significant fall of the regional blood flow. These hemodynamic changes are caused by increases of the regional and presumably also of the total peripheral vascular resistance. Most likely the increase in total peripheral vascular resistance represents an autoregulatory event triggered by the rising tissue oxygenation. From the present data it is difficult to estimate to what extent the observed rise in hematocrit affects peripheral vascular resistance also via an increase of blood viscosity.

References

1   Blumberg, A.: Die renale Anämie, pp. 99–126 (Huber, Bern 1972).

2   Böcker, A.; Reimers, E.; Nonnast-Daniel, B.; Kühn, K.; Koch, K. M.; Scigalla, P.; Braumann, K.-M.; Brunkhorst, R.; Böning, D.: Effect of erythropoietin treatment on O_2 affinity and performance in patients with renal anemia. Contr. Nephrol., vol. 66, pp. 165–175 (Karger, Basel 1988).

3   Bollinger, A.: Funktionelle Angiologie, pp. 1–25 (Thieme, Stuttgart, 1979).

4   Brod, J.; Fencl, V.; Hejl, Z.; Jirka, J.; Ulrych, M.: General and regional hemodynamic pattern underlying essential hypertension. Clin. Sci. 23: 339–349 (1962).

5   Casati, S.; Passerini, P.; Campise, M. R.; Graziani, G.; Cesana, B.; Perisic, M.; Ponticelli, C.: Benefits and risks of protracted treatment with human recombinant erythropoietin in patients having hemodialysis. Br. med. J. 295: 1017–1020 (1987).

6   Coleman, G.: Hemodynamics of uremia anemia. Circulation 45: 510–511 (1972).

7   Creutzig, A.; Dau, D.; Caspary, L.; Alexander, K.: Transcutaneous oxygen pressure measured at two different electrode core temperatures in healthy volunteers and patients with arterial occlusive disease. Int. J. Microcirc. 5: 373–380 (1987).

8   Cropp, G. J. A.; Hemodynamic responses to oxygen breathing in children with severe anemia. Circulation 40: 493–500 (1969).

9   Duling, B. R.; Berne, R. M.: Longitudinal gradients in periarteriolar oxygen tension: A possible mechanism for the participation of oxygen in local regulation of blood flow. Circulation Res. 27: 669–678 (1970).

10 Duling, B. R.; Pittman, R. N.: Oxygen tension: Dependent or independent variable in local control of blood flow? Fed. Proc. 34: 2012–2019 (1975).

11 Eschbach, J. W.; Egrie, J. C.; Adamson, J. W.: Correction of the anemia of end-stage renal disease with recombinant human erythropoietin results of a combined phase I and II clinical trial. New Engl. J. Med. 316: 73–78 (1987).

12 Graettinger, J. S.; Parsons, R. L.; Campbell, J. A.: A correlation of clinical and hemodynamic studies in patients with mild and severe anemia with and without congestive failure. Ann. intern. Med. 58: 617–625 (1963).

13 Levy, M. N.; Share, L.: The influence of erythrocyte concentration upon pressure/flow relation in dogs hind limb. Circulation Res. 1: 247–255 (1953).

14 Mitchell, T. R.; Pegrum, G. D.: The oxygen affinity of hemoglobin in chronic renal failure. Br. J. Haemat. 21: 463–472 (1971).

15 Neff, M. S.; Kim, K. E.; Persoff, M.; Onesti, G.; Swartz, C.: Hemodynamics of uremic anemia. Circulation 43: 876–883 (1971).

16 Pirofsky, B.: The determination of blood viscosity in man by a method based on Poiseuille's law. J. clin. Invest. 32: 292 (1953).

17 Rusch, E.; Sheppard, S. Welb, I.; Vanhautte, G.: Different behaviour of resistance vessels of calf and forearm in exercise and stress. Circulation Res. 48: 118–130 (1981).

18 Schmid-Schönbein, H.: Microrheology of erythrocytes, blood viscosity and distribution of blood flow in the microcirculation; in Messen, Handbuch der allgemeinen Pathologie, vol. 3, pp. 289–384 (Springer, Berlin 1977).

19 Whittaker, S.; Winton, F. R.: Apparent viscosity of blood flowing in isolated hind

limb of dog and variation with corpuscular concentration. J. Physiol. *78:* 339–369 (1933).

20 Winearls, C. G.; Pippard, M. J.; Downing, M. R.; Oliver, D. O.; Reid, C.; Cotes, M. P.: Effect of human erythropoietin derived from recombinant DNA on the anemia of patients maintained by chronic haemodialysis. Lancet *ii:* 1175–1177 (1986).

B. Nonnast-Daniel, MD, Department Innere Medizin und Dermatologie,
Abteilung Nephrologie, Medizinische Hochschule Hannover,
Konstanty-Gutschow-Strasse 8, D-3000 Hannover 61 (FRG)

Discussion

Bauer: I would like to congratulate you for this very nice paper, very nice data and a very nice presentation. That was my first point. The second point I want to make about the relationship between arteriolar diameter and pO_2. Despite the fact that there are certain people in the audience who would not believe in the importance of prostaglandins and their biological effects, it has been shown that this relationship is greatly blunted if one inhibits cyclooxygenase. This would indicate that part of the effects you see are due to the change in vascular tone, and not so much related perhaps to the change in viscosity when you increase hematocrit with EPO.

Schaefer (Würzburg): Just let me show you one slide. We actually did measurements of blood viscosity during treatment with EPO. Both plasma and whole blood viscosity were determined. As you can see, hemodialysis patients have an elevated plasma viscosity as compared to normal, healthy, sex- and age-matched subjects. During EPO treatment the value of plasma viscosity was unchanged. When we measured whole blood viscosity we found an increase during the rise of hematocrit values. However, at a hematocrit value of 35%, which represented our target hematocrit, whole blood viscosity was still lower as compared to normal subjects. Taken together, hemodialysis patients display an elevated plasma viscosity and if you increase the hematocrit values towards the normal range, you will have a rise in whole blood viscosity. Since whole blood viscosity is one of the determinants of peripheral resistance, this could represent one of the mechanisms which lead to higher blood pressure values in dialysis patients treated with recombinant EPO.

Baldamus: I have a question to both previous speakers concerning viscosity. Do you have any idea whether the flexibility and shape of erythrocytes changed, so that one could expect a change in viscosity which is hematocrit independent?

Schaefer: No, we did not look into that.

Koch: Dr. Schaefer, you saw our figures concerning the change of peripheral resistance. If you could make a quick calculation: Is the change of peripheral resistance we observed sufficiently explained by the change of viscosity you measured?

Schaefer: You saw a change of about plus 80%?

Nonnast-Daniel: Yes, an increase of about 80%.

Schaefer: If you use the changes of whole blood viscosity we measured, I calculate an increase of total peripheral resistance of approximately 40%.

Koch: So if the change of regional peripheral resistance Dr. Nonnast measured is representative for total peripheral resistance one has to postulate additional mechanisms to explain the rise in total peripheral resistance.

Bergström (Huddinge): I have a question to Dr. Nonnast. These data which suggest that it is a metabolic event which triggers the change in peripheral resistance are very interesting. I would like to know if you could elaborate on which factors could be of importance. Is it adenosine or some other factor?

Nonnast-Daniel: Our present data do not permit us to draw any conclusions concerning the nature of the vasoactive substances involved.

Bergström: So, what do you think it may be?

Nonnast-Daniel: I think it is an autoregulatory mechanism, but so far we do not know the substances involved. I do not think it is viscosity alone which causes the rise in peripheral resistance.

Nattermann: What is the optimum hematocrit? The cardiac output should not be too high, the peripheral resistance low and the viscosity not too high. So, is it perhaps 30 or is it 35%?

Nonnast-Daniel: I know from hemodilution studies in patients with occlusive arterial disease that one tries to reach a hematocrit value of 35%.

Nattermann: But I think this question must still be discussed as the aim of our therapy is to raise the hematocrit and to what level it should be raised?

Bauer: I think that is a very important question. There are two things to say about this. The optimum hematocrit is defined as the relationship between the product of cardiac output×hemoglobin concentration. The optimum hematocrit Richardson and Guyton found in animal experiments is in the 40% range. The normal hematocrit is around 40% and they found the optimum hematocrit just at this point. But this optimum hematocrit changes, because if the experimental animals are made anemic for a certain time, then the optimal hematocrit shifts towards lower values.

Nattermann: I know a paper by Hint published in *Acta Anesthesiology* Belgium in 1968. In acute anemia he showed that a hematocrit of 37% may be the best. There is another paper by Watkins, published in *Surgery of Gynecology and Obstetrics* in 1964 showing that in chronic anemia the cardiac output will increase at a hematocrit of 21%. These are two borders. Of course patients with a coronary heart disease need a higher hematocrit than normal patients. I think it is still difficult to have the right goal for hematocrit.

Bauer: I think the optimum hematocrit is not a fixed value. I mean that is what all these studies clearly show. The optimum hematocrit of around 40% might be true for normal people. But the moment one is getting chronically anemic, the optimum hematocrit shifts to lower values. One should not use a target hematocrit to evaluate EPO therapy but rather use functional tests, like step tests, because there is no such thing like an optimum hematocrit under all conditions.

Koch: A question to the physiologists: you referred a few times to the optimum hematocrit. What would be your definition of the optimum hematocrit?

Bauer: The definition of the optimum hematocrit is the point where the product of cardiac output × hemoglobin concentration is at a maximum. This would be the maximum oxygen flow per unit of time.

Koch: So, you based it on oxygen flow?

Bauer: That is right.

Creutzig: If you are looking at organ oxygenation, for instance muscle oxygenation, the optimum hematocrit seems to be in the range of 35%. There are experimental studies from Messmer in Heidelberg who could show in hemodilation that the muscle oxygenation increases when the hematocrit is lowered to 35 and decreases if the hematocrit is lowered below 35%.

Böning: There is a paper by Gaethgens in the *European Journal of Applied Physiology* (vol. 41, 1979) showing that the optimum hematocrit during exercise is higher than normal.

Contr. Nephrol., vol. 66, pp. 195–204 (Karger, Basel 1988)

Lymphocyte Subsets and Delayed Cutaneous Hypersensitivity in Hemodialysis Patients Receiving Recombinant Human Erythropoietin

W. Pfäffl[a], *H.-J. Gross*[b], *D. Neumeier*[b], *U. Nattermann*[a], *W. Samtleben*[a], *H. J. Gurland*[a]

[a]Nephrology Division, Medical Clinic I, and [b]Department of Clinical Chemistry, Klinikum München-Grosshadern, Ludwigs-Maximilians-University, München, FRG

Patients on long-term maintenance hemodialysis exhibit immunologic abnormalities due to depression of their cellular immune system. The reasons for this are not completely understood. This immunological defect manifests in their increased susceptibility to infections, prolonged allograft survival, lymphopenia and suppressed transformation of lymphocytes in response to mitogens, decreased delayed cutaneous hypersensitivity (DCH) or impaired B cell function to produce high titer antibody response [5, 6].

Recently, recombinant human erythropoietin (rhEPO) has become available and its efficacy in correcting renal anemia in patients on chronic hemodialysis has been shown [7, 8]. It is not clear if the improved physical condition and well-being in patients under rhEPO maintenance therapy is due only to an increased hematocrit or if it also reflects an improvement in some of their immunologic dysfunctions. Normalization of certain immune dysfunctions in chronic uremic patients would render them less susceptible to infections, but could have an adverse impact on the outcome of a subsequently transplanted allogenic graft. Furthermore, in vitro experiments show evidence that T lymphocytes consistently enhance the growth of peripheral blood erythroid burst-forming units (BFU-E) [1, 4], which are precursors of the differentiated normoblasts.

Since T lymphocytes modulate erythropoiesis, we monitored lymphocyte subsets and tested DCH in patients under rhEPO therapy. We inves-

tigated whether correction of renal anemia induces changes in the lymphocyte subsets or alters the response to different microbial recall antigens.

Materials and Methods

Study Design

Fifteen patients entered the study after having signed informed consent. The mean of
the age of the 13 female and 2 male patients was 55 years (range 23–74 years). Eight patients
suffered from end-stage glomerulonephritis, 3 from chronic pyeleonephritis, 2 from polycystic kidney disease, 1 from malignant hypertension and 1 from analgesic nephropathy.
All patients were more than 6 months on hemodialysis and suffered from renal anemia with
a hematocrit of less than 28 vol%. Patients were randomly subdivided into three groups,
which received 40, 80, or 120 U rhEPO/kg body weight three times a week intravenously
postdialysis until hematocrit had increased at least 10 vol% or had reached a maximum of
35 vol%. After this correction period, all patients received a standard maintenance dosage
of 15 U/kg body weight. This dose was increased weekly if hematocrit started to decrease.
To avoid interference with circadian changes in the white blood count and the influence of
the dialysis procedure, all blood samples were taken at the same time of the day and before
dialysis was started. Lymphocyte subpopulations were analyzed and DCH was tested at the
beginning of the study, after the correction of the renal anemia, and 18 weeks after start of
therapy with rhEPO (maintenance phase). Differential blood counts were obtained weekly.
Statistical comparisons were made by means of Student's paired t test. Statistically
significant differences were defined by a p value of less than 0.05. Results, if not otherwise
indicated, are expressed as means ± SD.

Flow Cytometry of Lymphocyte Subpopulations

Mononuclear cells were isolated from peripheral blood by Ficoll-Paque (Pharmacia,
Uppsala, Sweden) density centrifugation as described by Bøjum [9]. 250,000 cells were
stained with fluoresceinated monoclonal antibodies for 30 min at 4 °C. The following
monoclonal antibodies were applied: LEU4-FITC (CD3), LEU3-FITC (CD4), LEU2-FITC
(CD8), LEU12-FITC (CD19), HLA-DR-FITC and LEU7-FITC. After two washes with
phosphate-buffer saline 1% bovine serum albumin, the cells were analyzed by fluorescent-
activated cell sorter (FACS-STAR; Becton-Dickinson, Mountain View, Calif.).

DCH by Means of the Multitest System

The Multitest System (Mérieux, Lyon, France) test kit containing 0.03 ml of 7
standardized microbial recall antigens (tetanus toxoid, diphtheria toxoid, streptococcal
antigen, Tuberculin, Candida antigen, Trichophyton antigen and Proteus antigen) and 70%
glycerol as control was applied at the beginning of the study, after correction of renal
anemia, and after 18 weeks of maintenance therapy according to the manufacturer's
instructions. The Multitest System has been evaluated in 830 normal subjects (Institute
Mérieux) using a score that represents the sum in millimeters of the mean diameters of all
positive reactions. The recommended cut-off score to separate nonresponders from
responders is 5 mm for females and 10 mm for males. Since reactivity to the different
antigens may vary by age and sex, each patient was considered to be his own control.

Table I. Differential blood counts in 15 hemodialysis patients receiving rhEPO over a period of 18 weeks (mean ± SD)

	Prevalue	Initial phase	Maintenance
Leukocytes/μl	6,400 ± 1,500	6,200 ± 1,200	5,900 ± 900
Bands, %	0	0	0
Segmented, %	59,6 ± 8.4	63.5 ± 7.8	60.3 ± 11.0
Lymphocytes, %	26.5 ± 5.5	24.5 ± 7.1	25.8 ± 8.5
Eosinophils, %	4.5 ± 3.1	3.7 ± 3.0	4.7 ± 3.8
Basophils, %	0.5 ± 0.5	0.5 ± 0.6	0.9 ± 1.0

Results

In the 15 patients studied, the mean hematocrit significantly increased after initiation of rhEPO therapy from 22.3 ± 3.6 to 30.9 ± 2.7 vol% (p < 0.005) and stabilized after 18 weeks of therapy at a mean of 29.5 ± 2.9 vol% (p<0.005). The tendency to develop hypertension was the limiting factor preventing a further increase in hematocrit, which would be achievable by a prolonged maintenance of the rhEPO dosage in the correction period of hematocrit. Hypertension could be managed by reducing the weekly rhEPO dosage, or increasing antihypertensive medication and maintaining patients at an average hematocrit of 30 vol%.

Differential Blood Counts

All patients had normal white blood counts at the beginning of the study (mean 6,400 ± 1,500 mm^3), and these remained within the physiological range during the 18 weeks of the study. After 18 weeks of rhEPO therapy the mean leukocyte count had slightly decreased to 5,900 ± 900 mm^3 and was not significantly different from the mean leukocyte count obtained at the beginning of the study (table I). Differential blood counts did not show major deviations from the values obtained before rhEPO treatment was started. Lymphocytes represented 26.5 ± 5.5% of the differential blood count at the beginning of the study and were found to be 26.4 ± 8.5% after 18 weeks of rhEPO treatment (table I). No significant shifts in granulocytic cells were seen and these remained constant at around 60% of the differential blood count (table I). One patient, who was known to suffer from mild urticaria and itching during the dialysis procedure which could not be resolved by changing to different dialyzers, had a stable eosinophila of 15% throughout the study. Three other patients also had a persistent slight eosinophilia of up to 8%. No basophilia was seen during the 18 weeks of rhEPO treatment. Slightly elevated monocyte counts (mean $8.3 \pm 2.3\%$), as seen in some patients on long-term dialysis, persisted throughout the 18-week study period.

Lymphocyte Subpopulations

T cells (LEU4/CD3), normal range 730–2,240 cells/mm³: The absolute number of CD3-positive cells significantly decreased from $1,271 \pm 423$ cells/mm³ at the beginning of the study to $1,024 \pm 470$ cells/mm³ ($p < 0.01$) after 18 weeks of rhEPO therapy. The relative number of CD3-positive cells also significantly decreased from 76 ± 7 to $66 \pm 12\%$ ($p < 0.01$).

Helper cells (LEU3/CD4), normal range 440–1,540 cells/mm³: The absolute number of CD4-positive cells significantly decreased from 941 ± 363 to 751 ± 395 cells/mm³ ($p < 0.005$) after 18 weeks of rhEPO therapy. The relative number CD4-positive cells also significantly decreased from 56 ± 7 to $48 \pm 11\%$ ($p < 0.005$).

Suppressor cells (LEU2/CD8), normal range 190–920 cells/mm³: The absolute number of CD8-positive cells significantly decreased from 491 ± 203 cells/mm³ at the beginning of the study to 315 ± 159 cells/mm³ ($p < 0.005$) after 18 weeks of rhEPO therapy. The relative number of CD8-positive cells also significantly decreased from 30 ± 10 to $20 \pm 10\%$ ($p < 0.005$) during the study.

B cells (LEU12/CD19), normal range 87–260 cells/mm³: The absolute number of CD19-positive cells decreased from 169 ± 99 to 105 ± 74 cells/mm³ after the correction period but increased again to 208 ± 175 cells/mm³ after 18 weeks of rhEPO therapy. After 18 weeks no significant difference to the baseline value was noted. The relative number of B cells was significantly reduced after the initial period but returned to baseline levels after 18 weeks of rhEPO therapy (fig. 1).

Natural killer cells (LEU7): The absolute number of LEU7-positive cells decreased over a period of 18 weeks from 289 ± 189 to 215 ± 153 cells/mm³ ($p < 0.05$). The relative number of LEU7-positive cells decreased from 17.9 ± 11 to $15.3 \pm 10.5\%$. This decrease was not statistically significant.

Helper suppressor ratio (normal range 1.0–3.65): The relative number of CD8-positive cells decreased more than the relative number of CD4-positive cells resulting in a significant ($p < 0.05$) increase of the helper/suppressor cell ratio after 18 weeks (fig. 2).

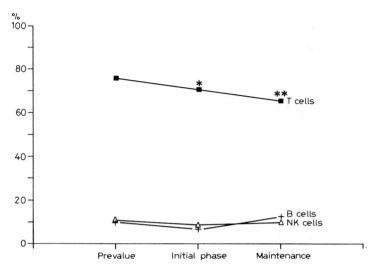

Fig. 1. Relative changes in the lymphocyte subpopulations of 15 patients receiving rhEPO over a period of 18 weeks (means, Student's paired t test: $^*p<0.05$; $^{**}p<0.01$).

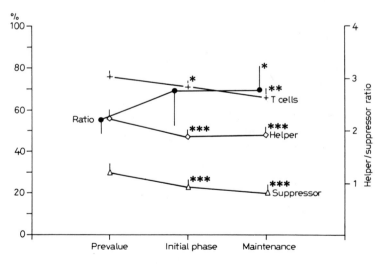

Fig. 2. Changes of lymphocyte subsets in 15 hemodialysis patients receiving rhEPO over a period of 18 weeks (means ± SEM, Student's paired t test: $^*p<0.05$; $^{**}p<0.01$; $^{***}p<0.005$).

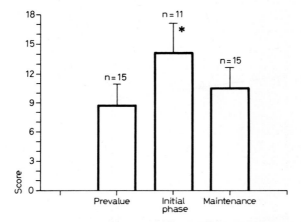

Fig. 3. Multitest System: Means ± SD of the DCH score in patients receiving rhEPO over a period of 18 weeks (see text for details). *p<0.05.

DCH (Multitest System): 6 of 13 female patients on maintenance hemodialysis demonstrated a score of more than 5 mm and were considered to be normoergic responders to the DCH test. The remaining 7 patients were considered hypo- or anergic with a score of less than 5 mm. The 2 male patients scored more than 10 mm and were considered to be normoergic. After correction of renal anemia, 11 of 15 patients were retested. Nine patients showed a transient rise in their DCH score. Two patients who were anergic at the beginning of the study did not improve their score. After 18 weeks of rhEPO therapy the DCH score in 11 patients did not differ from the score obtained at the beginning of the study. Four patients increased their DCH score to at least 5 mm. No significant decreases in DCH were observed (fig. 3).

Comments

We monitored lymphocyte subsets in 15 patients on maintenance hemodialysis who took part in a multicenter clinical study to prove efficacy of rhEPO and to find the adequate dosage for the correction of renal anemia. Significant changes in lymphocyte subpopulations were observed over an

18-week period. In the presence of an unchanged differential blood count, we observed a significant decrease in T cells while B cells increased. The decrease in the suppressor cell subpopulation was more pronounced than in the helper cell subpopulation resulting in a significant increase in the helper/suppressor cell ratio. These changes were apparent after the patients initially reached the maximum of their hematocrit and persisted when the patients were retested 18 weeks after start of rhEPO therapy.

Circadian variations of lymphocyte subsets are very well known [10–12]. Although the mechanism of these variations is not clear, different factors like the influence of hypothalamic hormones, intake of food, exercise, drugs or even emotional states have been discussed. Nothing is known about circadian variations of lymphocyte subsets in patients with end-stage kidney disease, but to avoid any influence of circadian rhythms or even the hemodialysis procedure, the blood samples were always taken at the same time of day before hemodialysis was started. It has to be taken into account that due to an increased incidence of hypertension in patients with corrected renal anemia [13], antihypertensive medication was changed in some of our patients. Most of our patients also reported an increased appetite and more physical activity while under rhEPO therapy.

Although we have observed phenotypic changes in the lymphocyte subpopulations, our study allows no conclusions on functional changes that might occur in patients under rhEPO therapy. Further studies, such as in vitro stimulation of lymphocytes from patients with and without rhEPO substitution will be necessary to show if functional changes also occur. Although chronic uremia induces certain general immune dysfunctions, our 15 patients suffered from five different underlying disease entities, which might all have different immunopathogenic backgrounds. More patients receiving rhEPO will have to be immunologically evaluated to separate the effects of a persistent underlying disease from the effects of rhEPO administration.

We also tested DCH in our patients while under rhEPO therapy. Seven out of 15 patients were anergic or showed a very low response to a defined set of recall antigens. This high incidence of decreased DCH is in accordance with the results of 253 patients on dialysis, which have been tested in our center [14]. In 7 of 11 patients retested at the end of the initial period, we noted a significant increase in their response to recall antigens. However, this returned to the level at the beginning of the study after 4 months of maintenance rhEPO therapy. The mean score of DCH of all patients was not significantly different from the mean of the prestudy score 18 weeks after rhEPO therapy, suggesting that underlying immunologic dysfunctions due to chronic uremia and hemodialysis persisted.

In this clinical experience with 15 patients under long-term rhEPO substitution therapy, we saw no evidence that the patients were less susceptible to infections. However, the significant changes in lymphocyte subpopulations observed during rhEPO therapy might have an impact on the outcome of a subsequent allogenic renal transplantation. For this reason we suggest immunological monitoring and further functional studies to evaluate the influence of rhEPO on the immune system.

References

1 Cline, M. J.; Golde, D. W.: Cellular interactions in hematopoiesis. Nature, Lond. *277:* 177–181 (1979).

2 Hamburger, A. W.: Enhancement of human erythroid progenitor cell growth conditioned by a human t-lymphocyte line. Blood *56:* 633–639 (1980).

3 Wisniewski, D.; Strife, A.; Wachter, M.; Clarkson, B.: Regulation of human peripheral blood erythroid burst-forming unit growth by T lymphocytes and T lymphocyte subpopulations defined by OKT4 and OKT8 monoclonal antibodies. Blood *65:* 456–463 (1985).

4 Lamperi, S.; Carozzi, S.: T lymphocytes, monocytes, and erythropoiesis disorders in chronic renal failure. Nephron *39:* 211–215 (1985).

5 Wilson, W. E. C.; Kirkpatrick, C. H.; Talmage, D. W.: Suppression of immunologic responsiveness in uremia. Ann. intern. Med. *62:* 1–14 (1965).

6 Goldblum, S. E.; Reed, W. P.: Host defenses and immunologic alterations with chronic hemodialysis. Ann. intern. Med. *93:* 597–613 (1980).

7 Eschbach, W. J.; Egrie, J. C.; Downing, M. R.; Browne, J. K.; Adamson, J. W.: Correction of the anemia of end-stage renal disease with recombinant human erythropoietin. New Engl. J. Med. *316:* 73–78 (1986).

8 Winearls, C. G.; Oliver, D. O.; Pippard, M. J.; Reid, C.; Downing, M. R.; Cotes, P. M.: Effect of human erythropoietin derived from recombinant DNA on the anemia of patients maintained by chronic hemodialysis. Lancet *ii:* 1175–1178 (1986).

9 Bøjum, A.: Isolation of mononuclear cells and granulocytes from human blood. Scand. J. clin. Lab. Invest. *21:* suppl., p. 99 (1977).

10 Berthouch, J. V.; Roberts-Thomson, P. J.; Bradley, J.: Diurnal variation of lymphocyte subsets identified by monoclonal antibodies. Br. med. J. *286:* 1171–1172 (1983).

11 Ferec, C.; Bourbigot, B.; Verlingue, C.; Airiau, J.; Deroff, P.; Saleun, J. P.: Circadian variations of lymphocyte subsets after renal transplantation. Transplant. Proc. *18:* 1308–1310 (1986).

12 Levi, F.; Canon, C.; Blum, J. P.; Reinberg, A.; Mathe, G.: Large amplitude circadian rhythm in helper:suppressor ratio of peripheral lymphocytes. Lancet *ii:* 462–463 (1983).

13   Samtleben, W.; Baldamus, C. A.; Bommer, J.; Fassbinder, W.; Nonnast-Daniel, B.;
     Gurland, H. J.: Blood pressure changes during treatment with recombinant human
     erythropoietin. Contr. Nephrol. vol. 66, pp. 114–122 (Karger, Basel 1988).
14   Stoffner, D.; Castro, L. A.; Habersetzer, R.; Hillebrand, G.; Drotleff, H.; Land, W.:
     Prognosis of cadaveric renal transplantation using a delayed cutaneous sensitivity test
     in dialysis patients. Transplant. Proc. 17: 2793–2794 (1985).

W. Pfäffl, MD, Department of Nephrology, Medical Clinic I, Klinikum
Grosshadern der Maximilians-Universität München, PO Box 702 260,
D-8000 München 70 (FRG)

Discussion

Bauer: The first statement you made in your summary suggests that there is a causal relationship between EPO and the lymphocyte subset. You suggest that EPO treatment has something to do with the changes of the lymphocyte subsets. In view of the fact that the subsets, as you told us, depend on so many variables that are not being controlled, it is difficult to assign a causal relationship with EPO.

Pfäffl: It is really hard to understand this phenomenon and I have to tell you that we were quite surprised about the significance levels we found in our group of patients. I think we need further studies to see what the clinical relevance of our observation is. I think that it is probably not a direct effect of erythropoietin because erythropoietin seems to act specifically on a certain cell at a certain stage of development of the normoblast. On the other hand, we are using quite significantly high levels of EPO to correct the renal anemia. There are, for instance, reports of T cell leukemias which also show a polycythemia. It can be speculated that at a very high dosage of EPO, the lymphocytes somehow get involved. But this is real speculation and we need much more data to put this on a strong basis.

Bauer: You told us just that these changes are highly significant. Am I right in assuming that you are talking about the statistical significance?

Pfäffl: Right.

Bauer: Now, what about the biological significance?

Pfäffl: The biological significance is to keep in mind that erythropoietin is a highly potent peptide which might have some effects we are not focusing on yet. We are observing so-called 'transients', you know, we are focusing on the things we are expecting anyway.

Bauer: What I mean is that there is no proven biological significance.

Pfäffl: If you look at the data: the helper/suppressor cell ratio goes up. This is significant, by the way. But it is still within the normal range. The helper cells and the suppressor cells, even if they go down significantly, are still in the normal range.

Varet: I can hardly understand how you can have a significant decrease in T lymphocytes without modification in the other subsets and in the total number of lymphocytes?

Pfäffl: This is very easy to understand when you consider that we count the absolute number of leukocytes first. Then we make a flow-cytometric analysis of the percentage of the subpopulations. From there we calculate back the absolute number of lymphocyte subsets. All the calculations of the absolute number of cells are based on the percentage of the total lymphocyte count.

Varet: What about the absolute numbers of T_8 and T_4 lymphocytes?

Pfäffl: The absolute number goes down. I showed you two slides.

Varet: Is this significant, too?

Pfäffl: Yes. We can look at these slides again. I showed you the absolute and relative changes.

Varet: Then you should have an increase in the absolute number of non-T-non-B lymphocytes.

Nielsen (Copenhagen): It might be of some interest to mention to you that we have checked the effect of recombinant EPO on the production of tumor necrosis factor and interleukin-1 by the macrophage and have found no effects so far. Just in terms of the effect of recombinant EPO on the immune system I wanted to add this comment.

Pfäffl: I think these data from 15 patients are not sufficient enough to make very strong conclusions yet. I have been looking in the literature for what is known about the effect of EPO on the T lymphocytes. There is really not much to be found. There is no clear data on whether there is a receptor on the T lymphocytes or whether a stimulation by erythropoietin is possible or not. We have very little evidence that this is a direct effect of erythropoietin. I think the changes of lymphocyte subsets are rather an effect of the corrected anemia than a direct effect of EPO.

Concluding Remarks

It is time to make a few concluding remarks. First of all I think we all agree that this has been a very successful meeting from the scientific point of view. The size of the meeting with around 70 participants is ideal to ensure good scientific communication and lively, stimulating discussions. The topic of the meeting 'Recombinant Erythropoietin' is one of the most interesting and challenging topics for the nephrologist today. Until now anemia has been one of the major unresolved medical problems in renal failure patients. Treatment with erythropoietin (EPO) should mean a major breakthrough for our patients with uremia by increasing physical work capacity, reducing fatigue and improving quality of life. Minimizing blood transfusions should prevent severe side effects such as viral infections (hepatitis, HIV), hemochromatosis and development of HLA antibodies which may minimize the chances of successful renal transplantation.

Concerning EPO there are still many questions unanswered and many problems awaiting a solution. For instance, we do not know exactly the role of erythropoietin for the development of hypertension. Furthermore, there are many questions about the metabolic effects of EPO which have to be solved. I am sure that we will have the opportunity to see each other again at several future meetings about EPO within the next few years.

We have all appreciated very much to have our workshop in Herzog August's Bibliothek in Wolfenbüttel. This Renaissance library is unique in the world and has conveyed to us a scientific tradition from many centuries ago.

On behalf of all of us I would like to thank Prof. Karl Koch and his co-workers who organized the meeting. Our gratitude goes especially to Dr.

Nonnast-Daniel, who has contributed so much to making this meeting a great success.

Last but not least I would like to express our gratitude to the Boehringer-Mannheim Company for sponsoring this meeting and for their generous hospitality.

Thank you very much.

Jonas Bergström

Subject Index